Medical Terminology

Jim Keogh, R.N.
Instructor, New York University

Schaum's Outline Series

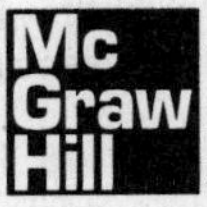

New York Chicago San Francisco Lisbon London Madrid
Mexico City Milan New Delhi San Juan Seoul
Singapore Sydney Toronto

The McGraw·Hill Companies

This book is dedicated to Anne, Sandy, Joanne, Amber-Leigh Christine, Shawn and Eric, without whose help and support this book couldn't have been written.

JIM KEOGH is a registered nurse and has written *Schaum's Outline of Pharmacology, Schaum's Outline of Nursing Laboratory and Diagnostic Tests, Schaum's Outline of Medical Charting,* and co-authored *Schaum's Outline of ECG Interpretation.* His books can be found in leading university libraries including Yale University School of Medicine, University of Pennsylvania Biomedical Library, Columbia University, Brown University, University of Medicine and Dentistry of New Jersey, Cambridge University, and Oxford University. Jim Keogh, RN, AAS, MBA, is a former member of the faculty at Columbia University and is a member of the faculty of New York University.

Schaum's Outline of
MEDICAL TERMINOLOGY

1 2 3 4 5 6 7 8 9 10 ROV/ROV 1 9 8 7 6 5 4 3 2 1

ISBN: 978-0-07-173652-7
MHID: 0-07-173652-2

Library of Congress Cataloging-in-Publication Data

Keogh, Jim, 1948- author.
Schaum's outline of medical terminology / James Keogh, R.N., Instructor, New York University.
p. ; cm. — (Schaum's outline series)
Outline of medical terminology
Summary: "This book provides a review of medical terminology for allied health and nursing students"—Provided by publisher.
ISBN-13: 978-0-07-173652-7 (alk. paper)
ISBN-10: 0-07-173652-2 (alk. paper)
ISBN-13: 978-0-07-173653-4 (e-book)
ISBN-10: 0-07-173653-0 (e-book)
1. Medicine—Terminology—Examinations, questions, etc. 2. Medicine—Terminology—Outlines,syllabi, etc. I. Title. II. Title: Outline of medical terminology.
[DNLM: 1. Terminology as Topic—Examination Questions. 2. Terminology as Topic—Outlines. W 18.2]

R123.K46 2011
610.1'4—dc22

2010047087

Contents

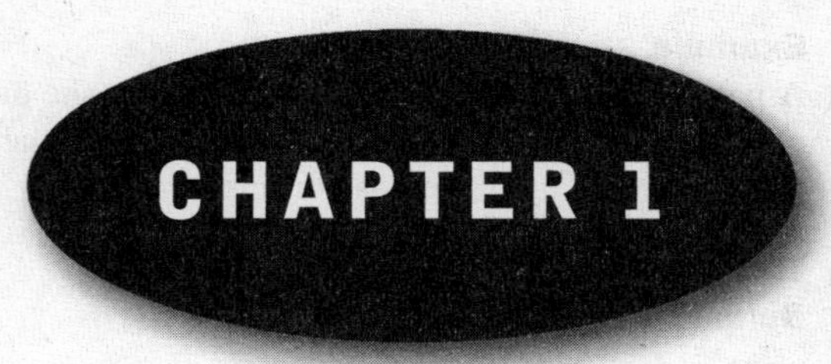

The Language of Medicine

1.1 Definition

At first, medical terminology might seem a foreign language that consists of long, hard-to-pronounce words that even health care providers sometimes have difficulty pronouncing. However, another way to think of medical terminology is like a secret message that becomes clear once you decode the message.

The first step in deciphering a medical term is to break it down into its components:

- **Root:** Each medical term has one or more roots that specify the subject of the term.
- **Suffix:** Each medical term has a suffix, which is the ending of the term that describes an aspect of the subject.
- **Vowel:** Most medical terms have a vowel whose sole purpose is to link the root and suffix. The vowel is usually an *o*.
- **Prefix:** Many medical terms have a prefix at the beginning of the term that modifies the root.
- **Combining Form:** The combining form is assembling the prefix, root, vowel, and suffix to form the medical term.

Reading a Medical Term

In order to read and understand a medical term, you need to learn the definitions of prefixes, roots, and suffixes, which you will learn through this chapter. Begin reading the medical term by identifying the root. The root usually identifies the part of the body. Next, read the suffix of the medical term. The suffix is at the end of the term and usually identifies the action. And then read the prefix of the medical term, if there is one. The prefix usually narrows the term to a particular aspect of the root.

Example: Epigastric

- **Root:** The root of epigastric is *gastr*. Think of *gastr* as the "code word" for stomach. Each time you see *gastr* in the medical term, you know that the term has something to do with the stomach.
- **Suffix:** The suffix of epigastric is *ic*. Think of *ic* as the "code word" for pertaining to something, which is usually the root. In this example, the medical term is pertaining to the stomach.
- **Prefix:** The prefix in epigastric is *epi*. Think of *epi* as the "code word" for above. Each time you see *epi* in the medical term, you know that term refers to above the root, which in this example refers to above the stomach.

Reading a Medical Term in a Sentence

Health care works translate nonmedical terms into medical terminology by finding the right combination of prefix, root, and suffix to create the combining form that specifically describes a medical situation.

Example

A patient tells the health care provider that she has burning pain slightly below her chest. After asking several questions to rule out problems with her heart, the health care provider will likely write in her chart: epigastric pain described by patient as burning.

Translation

Burning pain above the stomach.

1.2 Roots

The root of a medical term is either Greek or Latin and identifies the body part. Latin roots are joined to a suffix by an *o* such arthrology, which is the study of joints. However, the *o* is dropped when the suffix begins with a vowel such as arthritis, which is inflammation of a joint. Table 1.1 lists roots of medical terms and their definitions.

TABLE 1.1 Roots of Medical Terms

ROOT	DEFINITION
aden(o)	gland
adip	fat
allic	big toe
angi(o)	blood vessel
aort(o)	aorta
arteri(o)	artery
aur	ear
axill	armpit
balan(o)	glans/clitoridis penis
blephar(o)	eyelid
brachi(o)	arm
bronchi	bronchial tubes
bucc	cheek
capill	hair
capit(o)	head
cardi(o)	heart
carp(o)	wrist
cel	tumor
cephal(o)	head
cerat(o)	horn
cerebr(o)	brain
cervic	neck
cheil(o); chil(o)	lip
cheir(o); chir(o)	hand

ROOT	DEFINITION
cholecyst(o)	gallbladder
cili	eyelid
colo	colon
colp(o)	vagina
cor	pupil of the eye
cordi	heart
core; coro	pupil of the eye
cornu	horn
corpor	body
cost(o)	rib
cox	hip
crani(o)	skull
cut; cuticul	skin
cyst(o)	bladder
cyte	cell
dactyl(o)	finger; toe
dent(i)	tooth
derm; dermat(o)	skin
digit	finger; toe
dors	back
encephal(o)	brain
enter(o)	intestine
episi(o)	pubic region; vulva
faci(o)	face
fell	gallbladder
front(o)	forehead
gastr(o)	stomach
genu	knee
gingiv	gums
gloss; glott	tongue
gnath(o)	jaw
gon	knee
gon(o)	genitals
haem; haemat (foreign)	blood
hem; hemat	blood
hepat(o); hepatic	liver
humer(o)	shoulder

(Continued)

TABLE 1.1 Roots of Medical Terms (*Continued*)

ROOT	DEFINITION
hyster(o)	uterus; womb
jecor	liver
labi(o)	lip
lapar(o)	abdomen
laryng(o)	voice box/throat
lingu(a)	tongue
lip(o)	fat
mamm(o)	chest
mammill	nipple
manu	hand
mast(o)	breast
medull	bone marrow
ment	mind
metr(o)	uterus; womb
my(o)	muscle
myel(o)	bone marrow
nas	nose
nephr(o)	kidney
nerv; neur(o)	nerve
ocul(o)	eye
odont(o)	tooth
om(o)	shoulder
omphal(o)	navel
onc(o)	tumor
onych(o)	nail
oo	eggs
oophor(o)	ovary
ophthalm(o); optic(o)	eye
or	mouth
orchi(o); orchid(o)	testis
ossi; oste(o)	bone
ot(o)	ear
ov; ova	eggs
ovari(o)	ovary
palpebr	eyelid
papill	nipple
pe(o)	penis
pelv(i)	pelvis
phall(o)	genitals

ROOT	DEFINITION
pharyng(o)	throat
phleb(o)	vein
pleur(o)	rib
pneumon	lungs
pollic	thumb
psych	mind
pudend	pubic region
pulmo; pulmon(i)	lungs
pyel(o)	pelvis
pyret	fever
ren	kidney
rhin(o)	nose
salping(o)	fallopian tubes
sangui; sanguine	blood
sarping(o)	uterine tubes
sinus	sinus
som; somat	body
steth(o)	chest
stomat(o)	mouth
thele	nipple
thorac(i); thorac(o)	rib cage
thromb(o)	blood clot
trachel(o)	neck
trich(o)	hair
tum	tumor
umbilic	navel
ungui	nail
ur(o)	urinary system
ureter(o); urethr(a)	ureter
urethr(o)	urethra
urin(o)	urinary system
uter(o)	uterus; womb
vagin	vagina
vas; vascul	blood vessel
ven	vein
ventr(o)	stomach
vesic(o)	bladder
vulv	vulva

Roots followed by a vowel are commonly used to join the root with a suffix.

1.3 Prefixes

A prefix is located at the beginning of the medical term before the root. The function of the prefix is to further describe the root. For example, *cardia* is the root that refers to the heart. The prefix *brady* means slow. Therefore, the medical term bradycardia means a slow heart; that is, a heart rate slower than 60 beats per second. Some prefixes are joined to the root by a vowel. Table 1.2 lists common medical prefixes and their definitions.

TABLE 1.2 Common Medical Prefixes and Their Definitions

PREFIX	DEFINITION
a	absence of
ab	away from
abdomin(o)	relating to the abdomen
ac	sharp
acanth(o)	thorn or spine
acous(i, o)	relating to hearing
acr(o)	extremity; topmost
ad	adherence; increase; motion toward; very
aden(i, o)	relating to a gland
adip(o)	relating to fat or fatty tissue
adren(o)	relating to adrenal glands
aer(o)	air, gas
aesthesio	sensation
alb	white
alg(i, o); alge(si)	pain
allo	something different or addition
ambi	positioned on both sides or both of two
amnio	pertaining to the membranous fetal sac
an	absence of; not; without
an(o)	anus
ana	back; again; up
ancyl(o)	crooked or bent
andr(o)	pertaining to a man
angi(o)	blood vessel
angust(i)	narrow
aniso	unequal
ankyl(o)	bent; crooked
ante	positioned in front of another thing
anti	opposed to another
apo	derived from; separated from

PREFIX	DEFINITION
arch(i, e, o)	first; primitive
arseno	male; masculine
arteri(o)	pertaining to an artery
arthr(o)	pertaining to the joints; limbs
articul(o)	joint
atel(o)	imperfect or incomplete development
atri(o)	an atrium (esp. heart atrium)
aur(i)	pertaining to the ear
aut(o)	self
aux(o)	growth; increase
axill	pertaining to the armpit
azo(to)	nitrogenous compound
balano	pertaining to the glans clitoridis/penis
bar(o)	heavy
ben(e)	good; well
bi	double; twice
bio	life
bis	twice
blast(o)	germ or bud
blephar(o)	pertaining to the eyelid
bon(i)	good; well
brachi(o)	relating to the arm
brachy	short
brady	slow
brev(i)	short
bronch(i)	bronchus
bucc(o)	pertaining to the cheek
burs(o)	bursa
cac(o)	bad; incorrect
capill	pertaining to hair
capit	pertaining to the head
carcin(o)	cancer
cardi(o)	pertaining to the heart
carp(o)	pertaining to the wrist
cata	down; under
cav	hollow
celer	fast

(Continued)

TABLE 1.2 Common Medical Prefixes and Their Definitions (*Continued*)

PREFIX	DEFINITION
cephal(o)	pertaining to the head
cerat(o)	pertaining to the cornu (horn-shaped)
cerebell(o)	pertaining to the cerebellum
cerebr(o)	pertaining to the brain
cervic	pertaining to the cervix; neck
cheir(o)	pertaining to the hand
chem(o)	chemistry; drug
chir(o)	pertaining to the hand
chlor(o)	green
chol(e)	pertaining to bile
cholecyst(o)	pertaining to the gallbladder
chondr(i, o)	cartilage; gristle; granular; granule
chrom(ato)	color
cili	pertaining to the cilia; eyelashes; eyelids
circum	around; surrounding
cirrh(o)	red-yellow
cis	on this side
clast	break
co	in association; together; with
coel(o)	hollow
col(o); colono	colon
colp(o)	pertaining to the vagina
com	together; with
contra	against
cor; cor(e); coro	pertaining to eye's pupil; together; with
cordi	pertaining to the heart *(uncommon as a prefix)*
cornu	likened to horns
cost(o)	pertaining to the ribs
cox	relating to the haunch; hip; or hip joint
crani(o)	relating to the cranium
crass(i)	thick
cry(o)	cold
cutane	skin
cyan; cyan(o)	blue
cycl	circle; cycle

PREFIX	DEFINITION
cyph(o)	bent
cyst(i, o)	pertaining to the urinary bladder
cyt(o)	cell
dacryo	tear
dactyl(o)	pertaining to a finger or toe
de	away from; cessation
demi	half
dent-	pertaining to teeth
derm(o); dermat(o)	pertaining to the skin
dexi(o); dextr(o)	right
di(a)	apart; separation; two
dif	apart; separation
digit	pertaining to the finger
diplo	double
dis	separation; taking apart; twice
dors(i, o)	pertaining to the back
duodeno	pertaining to the duodenum
dupli	double
dur(i)	hard
dynam(o)	energy; force; power
dys	bad; difficult, incorrect
ec	away; out
ect(o)	outer; outside
encephal(o)	pertaining to the brain
endo	inside
enter(o)	of; pertaining to the intestine
epi	above
episi(o)	pertaining to the pubic region
equ(i)	equal
erythr(o)	red
esthesio	sensation
eu	good; new; true; well
eury	broad; wide
ex	away from; out of
exo	outside another
extra	outside
faci(o)	pertaining to the face

(Continued)

TABLE 1.2 Common Medical Prefixes and Their Definitions (*Continued*)

PREFIX	DEFINITION
fals(i)	false
fibr(o)	fiber
filli	fine; hairlike
flav	yellow
frig	cold
front	pertaining to the forehead
galact(o)	milk
gastr(o)	pertaining to the stomach
genu	pertaining to the knee
gingiv	pertaining to the gums
glauc(o)	bluish-gray
gloss(o); glott(o)	pertaining to the tongue
gluco	glucose
glyco	sugar
gnath(o)	pertaining to the jaw
gon(o)	pertaining to reproduction, seed, semen
grav(i)	heavy
gyn(aec, ec, o)	woman
haem; haemato; (foreign)	pertaining to blood
halluc	to wander in mind
hem; hema; hemat	pertaining to blood
hemi	half
hemo	blood
hepat; hepatic	pertaining to the liver
heter(o)	an addition or different
hidr(o)	sweat
hist(o); histio	tissue
hom(o)	the same
home(o)	similar
humer(o)	pertaining to the shoulder
hydr(o)	water
hyp(o)	below normal
hyper	extreme
hyster(o)	pertaining to the uterus; the womb
iatr(o)	pertaining to medicine
idio	one's own; self

PREFIX	DEFINITION
ileo	ileum
infra	below
inter	among; between
intra	within
irid(o)	iris
is(o)	equal
isch	restriction
ischio	pertaining to the hip joint
iso	equal
jaun	yellow
karyo	nucleus
kerat(o)	cornea
kin(e, o); kinesi(o)	movement
koil(o)	hollow
kyph(o)	humped
labi(o)	pertaining to the lip
lacrim(o)	tear
lact(i, o)	milk
laev(o)	left
lapar(o)	pertaining to the abdomen wall
laryng(o)	pertaining to the larynx
lat(i)	broad; wide
latero	lateral
lei(o)	smooth
lept(o)	light; slender
leuc(o); leuk(o)	white
levo	left
lingu(a, o)	pertaining to the tongue
lip(o)	fat
lith(o)	calculus; stone
log(o)	speech
lymph(a, o)	lymph/lymph node
lys(o)	dissolution
macr(o)	large; long
magn(i)	big; great; huge; large
mal(e)	bad; incorrect
malac(o)	soft

(Continued)

TABLE 1.2 Common Medical Prefixes and Their Definitions (*Continued*)

PREFIX	DEFINITION
mamm(o)	pertaining to the breast
mammill(o)	pertaining to the nipple
manu	pertaining to the hand
mast(o)	pertaining to the breast
maxim	biggest; largest
medi	middle
meg(a); megal(o)	enlargement; big; great; huge; large
megist	biggest; largest
melan(o)	black; denoting a black color
mening(o)	membrane
mero	part
mes(o)	middle
meta	after; behind
metr(o)	pertaining the uterus
micr(o)	small
minim	smallest
moll(i)	soft
mon(o)	single
morph(o)	form; shape
mort	dead
multi	many; much
muscul(o)	muscle
my(o)	relating to muscle
myc(o)	fungus
myel(o)	relating to bone marrow
myring(o)	eardrum
myx(o)	mucus
narc(o)	numb; sleep
nas(o)	pertaining to the nose
necr(o)	dead/death
neo	new
nephr(o)	pertaining to the kidney
nerv; neur(i, o)	pertaining to the nervous system
nigr	black
normo	normal
nov(i)	new
ocul(o)	pertaining to the eye
odont(o)	pertaining to teeth
odyn(o)	pain
ole	small or little
olig(o)	few

PREFIX	DEFINITION
om(o)	pertaining to the shoulder
omphal(o)	pertaining to the umbilicus
onco	bulk; tumor; volume
onych(o)	pertaining to the nail of a finger or toe
oo	pertaining to the ovum
oophor(o)	pertaining to the ovary
ophthalm(o)	pertaining to the eye
optic(o)	relating to chemical properties of the eye
or(o)	pertaining to the mouth
orchi(o); orchido	testis
orth(o)	correct; normal; straight
osseo	bony
ossi; ost(e); oste(o)	bone
ot(o)	pertaining to the ear
ov(i, o)	pertaining to the ovum
ovari(o)	pertaining to the ovaries
oxo	addition of oxygen
oxy	acid; acute; oxygen; sharp
pachy	thick
paleo	old
palpebr	pertaining to the eyelid
pan; pant(o)	complete
papill	pertaining to the nipple
papul(o)	a small elevation
para	abnormal; alongside of
parv(i)	small
path(o)	disease
pauci	few
ped	pertaining to the foot
pelv(i, o)	hip bone
peo	pertaining to the penis
per	through
peri	surrounding
pes	pertaining to the foot
phaco	lens-shaped
phagist	feeds on
phallo	phallus
pharmaco	drug; medication
pharyng(o)	pertaining to the pharynx
phleb(o)	pertaining to veins
phob(o)	exaggerated fear; sensitivity
phon(o)	sound

(Continued)

TABLE 1.2 Common Medical Prefixes and Their Definitions (*Continued*)

PREFIX	DEFINITION
phos; phot(o)	pertaining to light
phren(i, o); phrenico	diaphragm
plan(i); platy	flat
pleur(a, o)	pertaining to the ribs
pneum(o)	pertaining to the lungs
pneumat(o)	air, lung
pod	pertaining to the foot
poikilo	varied
polio	gray
poly	many
por(o)	porous
porphyr(o)	purple
post	after
prav(i)	bent; crooked
pre	before
presby(o)	old age
prim	most important
pro	before
proct(o)	anus; rectum
prot(o)	most important
pseud(o)	false
psych(e, o)	pertaining to the mind
pulmo; pulmon	relating to the lungs
purpur; purpureo	purple
pyel(o)	pelvis
pyo	pus
pyro	fever
quadr(i)	four
radio	radiation
re	again; backward
rect(i, o)	correct; straight; normal; rectum
ren(o)	pertaining to the kidney
reticul(o)	net
retro	backward; behind
rhabd(o)	rod-shaped; striated
rhachi(o)	spine
rhin(o)	pertaining to the nose
rhod(o); rub; rubr(o)	red
salping(o)	pertaining to the fallopian tubes
sangui; sanguine	pertaining to blood
sarco	fleshlike; muscular

PREFIX	DEFINITION
schist(o)	cleft; split
schiz(o)	split
scler(o)	hard
scoli(o)	twisted
semi	half
sial(o)	saliva; salivary gland
sigmoid(o)	sigmoid; sigmoid colon
sinistr(o)	left
sinus	pertaining to the sinus
sito	food; grain
somat(o); somatico	body; bodily
spasmo	spasm
sperma; spermato; spermo	semen, spermatozoa
splanchn(i, o)	viscera
splen(o)	spleen
spondyl(o)	pertaining to the spine
squamos(o)	full of scales
sten(o)	narrow
steth(o)	pertaining to the upper chest
stheno	strength; force; power
stom(a); stomat(o)	pertaining to the mouth
sub	beneath
super; supra	above; in excess; superior
sy(l); sym; syn; sys	likeness
tachy	fast
tard(i)	slow
thel(e, o)	pertaining to a nipple
thely	female
therm(o)	heat
thorac(i, o)	pertaining to the upper chest
thromb(o)	relating to a blood clot
thyr(o)	thyroid
toco	childbirth
tono	tension; tone; pressure
top(o)	place; topical
tox(i, o); toxico	poison; toxin
trache(o)	trachea
trachel(o)	pertaining to the neck
trans	something as moving
trich(i, o); trichia	pertaining to hairlike structure
tympan(o)	eardrum
ultra	beyond; excessive
umbilic	pertaining to the umbilicus
un(i)	one

(Continued)

TABLE 1.2 Common Medical Prefixes and Their Definitions (*Continued*)

PREFIX	DEFINITION
ungui	pertaining to the nail
ur(o)	pertaining to the urinary system
uri(c); urico	uric acid
urin	pertaining to the urinary system
uter(o)	pertaining to the uterus or womb
vagin	pertaining to the vagina
vari	varied; various
varic(o)	swollen or twisted vein
vas(o); vasculo	blood vessel; duct
ven	pertaining to veins
ventr(o)	pertaining to the stomach
vesic(o)	pertaining to the bladder
veter	old
vir	male; masculine; green
viscer(o)	pertaining to the internal organs
xanth(o)	yellow
xen(o)	different; foreign
zo(o)	animal; animal life
zym(o)	enzyme; fermentation

Prefixes are followed by a vowel used to join the prefix to the root.

1.4 Suffixes

The suffix follows the root or the vowel that connects the root to the suffix in a medical term. The suffix further describes the root. For example, the suffix in the medical term *hysterectomy* is *ectomy,* which is the removal of something. *Hyster* is the root that refers to womb. Therefore, hysterectomy is the removal of the womb, which is the uterus. Table 1.3 contains a list of suffixes used in medical terminology.

TABLE 1.3 Suffixes Used in Medical Terminology

SUFFIX	DEFINITION
ac	pertaining to
acusis	hearing
ad	in the direction of; toward
aemia	blood condition
al	pertaining to
algia	pain
ary	pertaining to
ase	enzyme
asthenia	weakness
ation	process

SUFFIX	DEFINITION
cele	hernia; pouching
centesis	surgical puncture for aspiration
cidal; cide	destroying; killing
crine	to secrete
cyte	cell
desis	binding
dynia	pain
eal	pertaining to
ectasis	dilation; expansion
ectomy	removal
emesis	vomiting condition
emia	blood condition
esophageal; esophago	gullet
form	having the form of
gen	born in; from
genic	pertaining to producing
gnosis	knowledge
gram; graph	record
graphy	process of recording
iasis	condition
iatry	a field in medicine
ic	pertaining to
icle	small
ics	organized knowledge; treatment
iform	having the form of
ism	condition; disease
ismus	contraction; spasm
ist	one who specializes in
ite	the nature of; resembling
itis	inflammation
ium	structure; tissue
lepsis; lepsy	attack; seizure
logist	a person who studies a certain field
logy	the study of a certain field
lysis	destruction
malacia	softening
megaly	enlargement
meter	measurement
metry	process of measuring
oid	resemblance to

(Continued)

TABLE 1.3 Suffixes Used in Medical Terminology (*Continued*)

SUFFIX	DEFINITION
ology	study of
oma; omata (pl.)	collection; mass; tumor
osis	condition; disease; increase
ous	pertaining to
paresis	slight paralysis
pathy	disease
penia	deficiency
pepsia	relating to digestion
pexy	fixation
phage; phagia	relating to eating
phago	devouring; eating
phagy	feeding on
phil(ia)	attraction for
plasia	formation
plasty	surgical repair
plegia	paralysis
plexy	stroke or seizure
poiesis	production
ptosis	drooping
ptysis	spitting
rrhage	burst forth
rrhagia	rapid flow of blood
rrhaphy	surgical suturing
rrhea; rrhoea	discharge; flowing
rrhexis	rupture
sclerosis	hardening of the skin
scope	instrument for viewing
scopy	use of instrument for viewing
sis	condition of
stasis	stop, stand
staxis	trickling
stomy	creation of an opening
tension; tensive	pressure
tic	pertaining to
tome	cutting instrument
tomy	cutting
tony	tension
tripsy	crushing
trophy	nourishment
ula; ule	small
y	condition or process of

Solved Problems

1.1 Interpret the term *cystotomy*.
cysto = bladder
tomy = cutting
cystotomy = an incision made into the urinary bladder

1.2 Interpret the term *bronchiectasis*.
bronchi = bronchial tubes
ectasis = dilation
bronchiectasis = dilation of the bronchial tubes

1.3 Interpret the term *erythrocyte*.
erythro = red
cyte = cell
erythrocyte = red cell (blood cell)

1.4 Interpret the term *hepatology*.
hepat = pertaining to the liver
ology = study of
hepatology = study of the liver

1.5 Interpret the term *intracranial*.
intra = within
crani = head
intracranial = within the head

1.6 Interpret the term *gingivitis*.
gingiv= gums
itis = inflammation
gingivitis = gum inflammation

1.7 Interpret the term *leukocyte*.
leuko = white
cyte = cell
leukocyte = white cell (blood cell)

1.8 Interpret the term *osteomalacia*.
osteo = bone
malacia = softening
osteomalacia = softening of bone

1.9 Interpret the term *metacarpus*.
meta = behind
carp = wrist
metacarpus = behind the wrist

1.10 Interpret the term *osteopenia*.
osteo = bone
penia = deficiency
osteopenia = bone deficiency

1.11 Interpret the term *phagocyte*.
phago = eating
cyte = cell
phagocyte = cell that eats other cells

1.12 Interpret the term *antipyretic*.
anti = against
pyret = fever
ic = pertaining to
antipyretic = against fever (medication)

1.13 Interpret the term *hypertension*.
hyper = extreme
tension = pressure
hypertension = extreme pressure (blood pressure)

1.14 Interpret the term *tachycardia*.
tachy = fast
cardia = heart
tachycardia = fast heart (heart rate above 100 beats per minute)

1.15 Interpret the term *tracheotomy*.
trache = neck
otomy = incision
tracheotomy= incision in the neck (windpipe)

1.16 Interpret the term *vaginitis*.
vagin = pertains to the vagina
itis = inflammation
vaginitis = inflammation of the vagina

1.17 Interpret the term *colostomy*.
colo = colon
stomy = opening
colostomy = opening in the colon

1.18 Interpret the term *spondylitis*.
spondyl = spine
itis = inflammation
spondylitis = inflammation of the spine

1.19 Interpret the term *salpingectomy*.
salping = fallopian tubes
ectomy = removal
salpingectomy = removal of the fallopian tubes

1.20 Interpret the term *hemorrhage*.
hem = blood
rrhage = bursting forward
hemorrhage = bursting forward blood (ruptured blood vessel)

1.21 Interpret the term *rhinoplasty*.
rhino = nose
plasty = surgical repair
rhinoplasty = surgical repair of the nose

1.22 Interpret the term *proctology*.
proct = anus; rectum
ology = study of
proctology = study of the anus/rectum

1.23 Interpret the term *dyspepsia*.
dys = bad; difficult; incorrect
pepsia = digestive tract
dyspepsia = difficulty digesting

1.24 Interpret the term *pachyderma*.
pachy = thick
derm = skin
pachyderma = thick skin

1.25 Interpret the term *onychophagia*.
onycho = nail
phagia = relating to eating
onychophagia = nail biting

Hematology Tests

2.1 Definition

Hematology is the study of blood, blood diseases, and organs that form blood. Hematology clinical laboratory tests are used to examine blood and blood components to determine if they are within normal limits. Values outside the normal limits might be indications of disease.

2.2 Blood Type .est

The blood type test is performed to test for blood compatibility for a blood transfusion and organ transplant and to test if a pregnant woman is Rh positive or negative.

Understanding the Blood Type Test

Blood is identified by antigens, which are specific proteins on the surface of red blood cells. There are two major types of antigens: blood group antigens (ABO) and Rh antigen. There are four types of blood group antigens that are determined by performing the ABO test:

1. **Type A:** Has the A antigen and antibodies in plasma against B antigen (Type B)
2. **Type B:** Has the B antigen and antibodies in plasma against A antigen (Type A)
3. **Type O:** Has neither the A antigen or the B antigen and antibodies in plasma against A antigen (Type A) and B antigen (Type B)
4. **Type AB:** Has the A antigen and the B antigen and no antibodies in plasma against A antigen (Type A) and B antigen (Type B)

Red blood cells may have the Rh antigen attached to their surface. This is sometimes referred to as the Rh factor and it is determined by the Rh test.

- Rh Positive (+): The Rh antigen is present on the red blood cells.
- Rh Negative (−): The Rh antigen is not present on the red blood cells.

A patient's blood type is described as a combination of blood group antigen and Rh antigen by using the blood type letter(s) followed by a plus (+) or minus (−) sign indicating if the Rh antigen is present. For example, Type A– means that the patient has the A antigen but does not have the Rh antigen attached to the red blood cells. The test also examines minor antigens that can cause an adverse blood transfusion reaction when attached to red blood cells.

2.3 Partial Thromboplastin Time (PTT) Test

The partial thromboplastin time (PTT) test assesses the blood's ability to clot, and is commonly performed before any invasive procedure. The PTT test is also used to measure the effectiveness of the dose of heparin administered to patients to prevent the formation of blood clots. This test is also used to assess for hemophilia and lupus anticoagulant syndrome or antiphospholipid antibody syndrome caused when the antibodies attack blood clotting factors.

Understanding the Partial Thromboplastin Time Test

When bleeding occurs, a cascade of 12 blood clotting factors is activated that causes the blood to coagulate to stop the bleeding. Coagulation of blood is affected by blood clotting factors. Their levels can be absent, decreased, or increased, as well as changes in the way blood clotting factors function. In addition, clotting inhibitors can reduce the effectiveness of clotting factors. The PTT test measures clotting time of blood.

Other blood clotting tests are prothrombin time (PT) and activated partial thromboplastin time (APTT). The heparin neutralization assay is performed to determine if substances other than heparin cause an increase in APTT.

2.4 Total Serum Protein Test

The total serum protein test is performed to assess for liver and kidney function (albumin); malnutrition (albumin); and the cause of edema, ascites, and pulmonary edema (albumin). It is also administered to assess for the risk for infection (globulin), multiple myeloma (globulin), and macroglobulinemia (globulin).

Understanding the Total Serum Protein Test

The total serum protein test assesses the levels of albumin, globulin, and total protein in a blood sample. The result compares the ratio of albumin to globulin. Protein is not stored. It is continuously metabolized into amino acids, which are used to make enzymes, hormones, and new proteins.

- **Albumin:** A protein produced by the liver that keeps blood from leaking from blood vessels. Albumin is also important for tissue growth and healing because it carries medicine to tissues.
- **Globulin:** A group of proteins made by the liver and the immune system that binds with hemoglobin and transports iron and metals in the blood to help fight infection. Globulin is composed of three different proteins: alpha, beta, and gamma.

A test for total serum protein reports separate values for total protein, albumin, and globulin. The amounts of albumin and globulin also are compared (albumin: globulin ratio).

2.5 Blood Alcohol Test

The blood alcohol test is administered to screen for intoxication, ingested alcohol, and the underlying cause of altered mental status.

Understanding the Blood Alcohol Test

Alcohol depresses the central nervous system (CNS) when large amounts of alcohol enter the blood. Alcohol is absorbed within a few minutes and peaks within an hour. Food decreases alcohol absorption. Alcohol is mostly metabolized by the liver and excreted in urine and by expiration. The blood alcohol test measures the level of alcohol in the blood.

The patient's signed consent may be required before the test is administered because the result of the blood alcohol test can have legal repercussions for the patient. Consult the health care facility's policies regarding administering the blood alcohol test.

A taximeter that measures alcohol levels in the patient's breath is another test to determine the level of alcohol consumed by the patient.

2.6 Lead Test

The lead test is administered to screen for lead poisoning and assess the treatment of lead poisoning.

Understanding the Lead Test

Lead affects growth and development if it is ingested via tainted water, paint chips, food, or dust particles or if lead comes in contact with the skin. Pregnant women can pass lead to the fetus or the newborn through breast milk. Children who are in early development are at risk for permanent growth impairment if they ingest lead. The lead blood test measures the level of lead in the blood sample.

The health care provider may order the urine aminolevulinic acid (ALA) test to determine the extent of lead poisoning (not for children). The lead mobilization urine test is performed during chelation therapy to assess if the therapy is removing lead in urine.

2.7 Serum Osmolality Test

The serum osmolality test is performed to screen for dehydration, overhydration, the underlying cause of seizure and coma, and the syndrome of inappropriate secretion of antidiuretic hormone (SIADH); and to assess the quantity of poison ingested by the patient.

Understanding the Serum Osmolality Test

Serum osmolality is the number of particles of substances that are dissolved in the serum (liquid). These substances include glucose, chloride, sodium, proteins, and bicarbonate. Serum osmolality balance is maintained between the ratio (or proportion) of fluid and particles of substances.

Serum osmolality is controlled by adjusting the fluid output of the kidneys using the antidiuretic hormone (ADH) produced by the pituitary gland. ADH is a vasopressin that reduces fluid output from the kidneys when ADH is released into the bloodstream, thereby increasing fluid in the blood. A decrease in ADH production increases fluid output by the kidneys and decreases fluid in the blood.

A decrease in fluid results in an increase in serum osmolality, or less fluid in the blood. This condition signals the pituitary gland to release ADH, which stimulates the kidneys to retain fluid, thereby increasing fluid in the blood and decreasing serum osmolality–fluid level in the blood is restored.

An increase in fluid results in a decrease in serum osmolality, or more fluid in the blood. This signals the pituitary gland to stop releasing ADH, which causes the kidneys to increase the output of fluid, thereby decreasing fluid in the blood and increasing serum osmolality–fluid level in the blood is restored.

The serum osmolality test measures the amount of substances dissolved in blood.

The health care provider may test urine osmolality. The result of the urine test is compared with the serum osmolality to estimate kidney function.

2.8 Uric Acid Blood Test

The uric acid blood test is performed to screen for uric acid kidney stones, gout, and adverse reaction of radiation therapy and chemotherapy. It is also used to assess treatment for hyperuricemia.

Understanding the Uric Acid Blood Test

Uric acid is produced when purine, which is contained in some foods, is metabolized. Uric acid enters the blood and is then excreted by the kidneys in urine and a small amount in stool. The uric acid test measures the level of uric acid in blood. The health care provider may order a 24-hour uric acid urine test.

Uric crystals can form in joints leading to gout even when uric acid levels are normal. A high level of uric acid does not mean that the patient has gout. Gout is diagnosed by testing fluid from the affected joint for uric acid crystals.

2.9 C-Reactive Protein (CRP) Test

The C-reactive protein (CRP) test is performed to screen for inflammation, assess for the effects of an intervention in the treatment of inflammation, screen for diseases that cause inflammation, and assess the patient's response to cancer treatment.

Understanding the C-Reactive Protein Test

C-reactive protein is produced as part of the inflammatory process and attaches to the invading microorganism or damaged cells, enhancing phagocytosis in the destruction of the microorganism or damaged cell. A high level of C-reactive protein indicates there is inflammation. Other tests are then performed to identify the source of the inflammation.

The high-sensitivity CRP test (hs-CRP) may also be ordered to determine if inflammation has damaged the inner lining of arteries, increasing the risk of a heart attack. In addition, the total cholesterol test and high-density lippoprotein (HDL) cholesterol test might be ordered with the C-reactive protein test to help determine if the patient is at risk for cardiac problems.

2.10 Complete Blood Count (CBC) Test

The complete blood count (CBC) test is performed to screen for anemia, infection, leukemia, the risk for bleeding, polycythemia, blood loss, asthma, allergies, and the underlying cause of bruising, and fatigue.

Understanding the Complete Blood Count Test

The CBC test, part of a routine blood screening, measures blood components to assess the patient for various disorders. The health care provider may also order the erythrocyte sedimentation rate (ESR) test to detect inflammation and the reticulocyte count to identify the number of immature leukocytes.

Here are the blood components that are measured:

- **Leukocyte Count (white blood cell count, WBC):** Leukocytes increase when infection is present and can also increase in the absence of infection if the patient has leukemia.
- **Leukocyte Cell Type (WBC differential):** There are five major types of leukocyte cells, each having a role in the immune process. These are *neutrophils, lymphocytes, monocytes, eosinophils,* and *basophils.* The quantity of each leukocyte cell type provides important information in the diagnoses of a patient's condition.
- **Erythrocyte Count (red blood cell count, RBC):** Erythrocyte cells carry oxygen and carbon dioxide.
- **Erythrocyte Indices:**
    - *Mean Corpuscular Volume (MCV):* This is the size of erythrocytes.
    - *Mean Corpuscular Hemoglobin (MCH):* This is the amount of hemoglobin in an erythrocyte cells.
    - *Mean Corpuscular Hemoglobin Concentration (MCHC):* This is concentration of hemoglobin in an erythrocyte cell.
    - *Red Cell Distribution Width (RDW):* This shows the different sizes of erythrocyte cells.

- **Hematocrit (HCT, packed cell volume):** The hematocrit test measures the volume in percentage taken up by erythrocytes in the patient's blood.
- **Hemoglobin (Hgb):** The hemoglobin test measures the amount of hemoglobin in blood. Hemoglobin is the part of an erythrocyte that carries oxygen.
- **Thrombocyte Count (platelet):** Platelets form blood clots.

2.11 Chemistry Screen Test

A chemistry screen test examines blood components and is used to assess the patient's overall health. The chemistry screen test is a collection of other tests that can include:

- Albumin
- Alkaline phosphatase
- Alanine aminotransferase (ALT)
- Aspartate aminotransferase (AST)
- Bilirubin
- Blood glucose
- Blood urea nitrogen
- Calcium (Ca) in blood
- Carbon dioxide
- Chloride (Cl)
- Cholesterol and triglycerides
- Creatinine and creatinine clearance
- Lactic acid
- Phosphate in blood
- Potassium (K) in blood
- Sodium (Na) in blood
- Total serum protein
- Uric acid in blood

Understanding the Chemistry Screen Test

There are various types of chemistry screen tests, including chem-20, chem-12, and chem-7. The number represents the number of blood components examined in the test.

A chemistry screen test is also called sequential multichannel autoanalysis (SMA) or sequential multichannel analysis with computer (SMAC) followed by the number of components being examined.

2.12 Vitamin B_{12} Test

The vitamin B_{12} test is performed to screen for vitamin B_{12} deficiency and for the underlying cause of anemia, peripheral neuropathy, and dementia.

Understanding the Vitamin B_{12} Test

Vitamin B_{12} is required for cell growth and metabolism and is stored in the liver. The vitamin B_{12} test measures the level of vitamin B_{12} in a blood sample. It is not unusual for the health care provider to order the folic acid test along with the vitamin B_{12} test and the Schilling test to assess the patient's ability to absorb vitamin B_{12}.

2.13 Cold Agglutinins Test

The cold agglutinins test is performed to screen for hemolytic anemia and the underlying cause for pneumonia.

Understanding the Cold Agglutinins Test

Agglutinins are antibodies that cause red blood cells to form a clump called rouleaux formation at low temperatures. This is an immune reaction to an infection. High levels of agglutinins can impede blood flow to the extremities when exposed to cold, resulting in tissue damage, and can cause hemolytic anemia. The cold agglutinins test measures the level of agglutinins in a blood sample.

2.14 Toxicology Tests (Tox Screen)

Toxicology tests are performed to screen for the use of medication (toxin), the underlying cause of the patient's unusual behavior, and the reason the patient is unconscious.

Understanding Toxicology Tests

A toxin is a substance that disrupts the body's function and includes prescription medication, nonprescription medication, and illegal medication. Toxicology tests measure the levels of one or a series of toxins in a blood sample. The health care provider may order a urine toxicology test, because traces of toxins can remain in urine longer than in blood, and a saliva toxicology test.

2.15 Folic Acid Test

The folic acid test is performed to screen for malnutrition, anemia, malabsorption, and assess the treatment of folic acid deficiency and the level of folic acid during pregnancy to reduce the risk of birth defects.

Understanding the Folic Acid Test

Folic acid, a type of vitamin B, is necessary for cell development and maintenance. Women who plan to become pregnant should increase the intake of folic acid to reduce the risk of spina bifida and cleft lip and palate. The folic acid test measures the level of folic acid in blood. The health care provider may order a vitamin B_{12} blood test along with the folic acid blood test.

2.16 Gastrin Test

The gastrin test is performed to screen for Zollinger-Ellison syndrome, pernicious anemia, pancreatic tumor, and G-cell hyperplasia.

Understanding the Gastrin Test

Gastrin is a hormone produced by the G cells of the stomach lining when food enters the stomach. Gastrin stimulates the parietal cells in the stomach to secrete hydrochloric acid (HCl) that is used in digestion and stimulates the product of pepsin, which is a digestive enzyme. The gastrin test measures the level of gastrin in the blood. The health care provider may order an intravenous secretin test where secretin, a digestive hormone, is injected into a vein and blood samples are taken immediately, then every 5 minutes for 15 minutes and then at 30 minutes.

2.17 Ferritin Test

The ferritin test is performed to screen for hemochromatosis (excess iron), iron deficiency anemia, and inflammation; and to assess for the effects of treatment of hemochromatosis and iron deficiency anemia.

Understanding the Ferritin Test

Ferritin is a protein found in bone marrow, liver, skeletal muscles, and the spleen that binds to iron. The ferritin test measures the level of ferritin in blood to determine the amount of iron in the body. Blood should contain a small amount of ferritin since most ferritin is bound to iron.

2.18 Lactic Acid Test

The lactic acid test is performed to screen for lactic acidosis, tissue oxygenation, and the underlying cause of acidosis.

Understanding the Lactic Acid Test

Muscle cells convert glucose into lactic acid and use lactic acid for energy when oxygen levels are low during strain of heart failure, exercise, shock, and sepsis. Lactic acid is not used for energy when there is a normal oxygen level in the blood. Lactic acid is metabolized by the liver. Liver disorders can result in lactic acidosis due to a high level of lactic acid in the blood. The lactic acid test measures the level of lactic acid in blood. The health care provider may order an arterial blood gas test to measure lactic acid in blood.

2.19 Prothrombin Time (PT) Test

The prothrombin time (PT) test is performed to screen for the risk for bleeding, bleeding disorders, vitamin K deficiency, and liver function, and to assess the therapeutic level of warfarin.

Understanding the Prothrombin Time Test

There are 12 factors that must be present and active to coagulate (clot) blood. Prothrombin is clotting factor II synthesized by the liver with the assistance of vitamin K. When a blood vessel is injured, prothrombin is converted to thrombin, a protein that forms a blood clot with other proteins to stop the bleeding. The PT test is the time necessary for plasma to clot. The health care provider orders the PT test to assess the patient's risk for bleeding and assess the therapeutic effect of anticoagulate medication.

The health care provider is likely to order the international normalized ratio (INR) test, which was established by the World Health Organization (WHO) as a standard for measuring blood coagulation. In addition, the health care provider is likely to order the PTT test to measure blood coagulation and the CBC to measure the platelet count.

2.20 Reticulocyte Count

The reticulyte count test is performed to screen for anemia and assess the treatment of anemia. It is also an indication of the bone marrow's response to the loss of RBCs, in which it produces new RBCs, known as reticulocytes.

Understanding the Reticulocyte Count

A reticulocyte is an immature red blood cell that is released by bone marrow and develops into a mature red blood cell in 2 days. The reticulocyte count test determines the amount of reticulocyte in a blood sample. The health care provider may order the reticulocyte index (RI).

2.21 Schilling Test

The Schilling test is performed to assess the absorption of vitamin B_{12} and the production of the intrinsic factor.

Understanding the Schilling Test

Vitamin B_{12} is the key to cell metabolism and energy production. Vitamin B_{12} attaches to the intrinsic factor produced by the parietal cells in the stomach. The intrinsic factor protects vitamin B_{12} from intestinal bacteria and enables absorption of vitamin B_{12} by the intestines. The Schilling test measures the absorption of vitamin B_{12}.

There are two parts to the Schilling test:

Part 1: The patient ingests vitamin B_{12} that is radioactively tagged. A 24-hour urine sample is examined for the presence of vitamin B_{12}. Up to 25% of the ingested vitamin B_{12} will normally be detected in the 24-hour urine sample. Little or no vitamin B_{12} detected is a sign of vitamin B_{12} malabsorption.

Part 2: If part 1 is abnormal, then the health care provider may order part 2. The patient ingests vitamin B_{12} that is radioactively tagged plus the intrinsic factor. A 24-hour urine sample is examined for the presence of vitamin B_{12}. Detection of vitamin B_{12} is a sign that the patient has pernicious anemia. Absence of vitamin B_{12} is a sign of an intestinal absorption problem.

The Schilling test is not performed on a pregnant woman or a woman who is breast-feeding. The health care provider may order a 48- or 72-hour urine sample if the patient has kidney disease. The health care provider may also order the methylmalonic acid (MMA) test and the homocysteine test.

2.22 Sedimentation Rate (SED) Test

The sedimentation rate (SED) test is performed to screen for inflammation and assess treatment for inflammation.

Understanding the Sedimentation Rate Test

An increase in fibrinogen in blood during the inflammatory process causes erythrocytes (RBC) to adhere to each other, forming a stack called rouleaux. The SED test measures how many millimeters per hour erythrocytes settle to the bottom of a test tube. Rouleaux settle quicker than erythrocytes; therefore, the increased SED indicates that the patient has inflammation. Not all inflammation increases the SED. Therefore, a normal SED does not rule out inflammation. The health care provider might order other tests (e.g., the CRP test) in addition to the SED to diagnosis inflammation.

2.23 Iron (Fe) Test

The iron (Fe) test is performed to screen for iron deficiency anemia or hemochromatosis, assess the nutritional status of the patient, and treat iron deficiency anemia.

Understanding the Iron Test

Iron is a mineral in food that is needed for cell growth. Once metabolized, iron binds to the transferrin protein, which transports iron to bone marrow and other tissues. The iron tests measure the amount of iron that is bound to transferrin.

There are three iron tests:

- **Total Iron Binding Capacity (TIBC) Test:** This test measures the capacity of the blood to carry iron by determining the amount of iron needed to bind to all the available transferring protein.

- **Serum Iron Test:** This test measures the amount of circulate iron in blood.
- **Transferrin Saturation Test:** This is the percentage of serum iron of total iron binding capacity.

The health care provider may order the ferritin test, the siderocyte stain test, and a CBC along with the iron tests.

2.24 Serum Protein Electrophoresis (SPE) Test

The serum protein electrophoresis (SPE) test is performed to screen for amyloidosis, multiple myeloma, and macroglobulinemia, and assess the underlying cause of hypogammaglobulinemia (HGG).

Understanding the Serum Protein Electrophoresis Test

Blood serum contains two groups of protein. These are albumin and globulin. Serum protein electrophoresis separates albumin and globulin into five groups by placing the sample of blood serum on an agarose gel and then exposing the gel to an electric current.

The five groups are:

1. Albumin
2. Alpha-1 globulin
3. Alpha-2 globulin
4. Beta globulin
5. Gamma globulin (antibodies)

Serum protein electrophoresis is not used to diagnose liver disorders, kidney disorders, or rheumatoid arthritis, although abnormal protein levels may be associated with these disorders. The health care provider may order urine protein electrophoresis. The health care provider may also order the total serum protein test along with the serum protein electrophoresis.

2.25 Arterial Blood Gases Test

The arterial blood gases test is performed to assess how well lungs exchange oxygen and carbon dioxide. In addition, measuring the oxygen saturation of the blood indicates the amount of hemoglobin that is carrying oxygen, and measuring the oxygen content of blood indicates the amount of oxygen in the blood.

This test assesses:

- Gas exchange capabilities of the lungs
- Effectiveness of treatment for lung disease
- Blood acidity level
- Effectiveness of treatment for an imbalance of blood acidity
- Kidney function

Understanding the Arterial Blood Gases Test

Blood contains oxygen and carbon dioxide. Measuring the partial pressure of these gases indicates how well lungs exchange oxygen and carbon dioxide. In addition, measuring the oxygen saturation of the blood indicates the amount of hemoglobin that is carrying oxygen, and measuring the oxygen content of blood indicates the amount of oxygen in the blood.

Blood must be within acidity range. Acidity is measured using the pH scale, which measures the hydrogen ions ($H+$). The pH of blood must be between 7.35 and 7.45 pH. If the measurement on the pH scale is <7.35, the blood is considered too acidic. If the measurement is >7.45, the blood is too alkaline (basic). Bicarbonate (HCO_3) is a chemical in the blood that ensures that the blood remains within the acceptable pH range. If blood becomes too acidic, the amount of bicarbonate is increased by increasing the absorption of bicarbonate by the kidneys.

2.26 Total Carbon Dioxide Test

The total carbon dioxide test measures the level of three types of carbon dioxide and is administered at the same time as the arterial blood gas test. The total carbon dioxide test is part of the chemistry screen.

The total carbon dioxide test assesses:

- Lung function
- Kidney function

Understanding the Total Carbon Dioxide Test

Carbon dioxide is a gaseous by-product of metabolism that is transported to the lungs where carbon dioxide is exhaled. Blood contains three forms of carbon dioxide. These are bicarbonate (HCO_3), carbonic acid (H_2CO_3), and dissolved carbon dioxide (CO_2). Most of the carbon dioxide is in the form of bicarbonate. Levels of these types of carbon dioxide are balanced by the lungs and kidneys.

2.27 Carbon Monoxide (CO) Test

The carbon monoxide (CO) blood test measures the level of carboxyhemoglobin in blood. The carbon monoxide blood test assesses:

- Exposure to breathing carbon monoxide
- Underlying symptoms of headache, dizziness, vision problem, muscle weakness, confusion, extreme sleepiness, and nausea or vomiting are caused by carbon monoxide

Understanding the Carbon Monoxide Test

Carbon monoxide is a colorless, odorless gas that replaces oxygen attached to the hemoglobin RBCs, creating a compound called carboxyhemoglobin that decreases oxygenation of blood and can result in death.

Solved Problems

Hematology Tests

2.1 What is the purpose of a blood type test?

Blood types tests are performed to test for blood compatibility for a blood transfusion and organ transplant, and to test if a pregnant woman is Rh positive or negative.

2.2 Why would a health care provider order a partial thromboplastin time (PTT) test?

The PTT test assesses the blood's ability to clot and is commonly performed prior to any invasive procedure. The PTT test is also used to measure the effectiveness of the dose of heparin administered to patients to prevent the formation of blood clots. This test is also used to assess for hemophilia and for lupus anticoagulant syndrome or antiphospholipid antibody syndrome, which are caused when the antibodies attack blood clotting factors.

2.3 What is the purpose of administering the total serum protein test?
The total serum protein test is given to assess for liver and kidney function (albumin), malnutrition (albumin), and the cause of edema, ascites, and pulmonary edema (albumin). It is also administered to assess for the risk of infection (globulin), multiple myeloma (globulin), and macroglobulinemia (globulin).

2.4 Why is the blood alcohol test ordered?
The blood alcohol test is administered to screen for intoxication, ingested alcohol, and for the underlying cause of altered mental status.

2.5 Name two reasons that a health care provider might order the lead test.
The lead test is administered to screen for lead poisoning and assess the treatment of lead poisoning.

2.6 What test would be ordered to assess for dehydration and overhydration?
The serum osmolality test would be ordered to assess for dehydration and overhydration.

2.7 What test might be ordered to assess the presence of the syndrome of inappropriate secretion of antidiuretic hormone (SIADH)?
The serum osmolality test might be ordered to assess the presence of SIADH.

2.8 Why would the uric acid blood test be ordered?
The test is performed to screen for uric acid kidney stones, gout, and adverse reaction of radiation therapy and chemotherapy. It is also used to assess treatment for hyperuricemia.

2.9 What is the purpose of the C-reactive protein (CRP) test?
The C-reactive protein (CRP) test is performed to screen for inflammation, assess the treatment for inflammation, screen for diseases that cause inflammation, and assess the patient's response to cancer treatment.

2.10 What might a high level of C-reactive protein indicate?
A high level of C-reactive protein (CRP) might indicate that there is inflammation.

2.11 What test is ordered to assess the risk for bleeding, infection, and the underlying cause of bruising and fatigue?
The complete blood count (CBC) test is ordered to assess the risk for bleeding, infection, and the underlying cause of bruising and fatigue.

2.12 What is the function of the chemistry screen test?
A chemistry screen test examines blood components and is used to assess the patient's overall health.

2.13 What test might be ordered to assess the underlying cause of anemia, peripheral neuropathy, and dementia?
The vitamin B_{12} test might be ordered to assess the underlying cause of anemia, peripheral neuropathy, and dementia.

2.14 Why would a health care provider order the cold agglutinins test?
The cold agglutinins test is performed to screen for hemolytic anemia and the underlying cause for pneumonia.

2.15 What test might a health care provider order if the patient displays unusual behavior and then becomes unconscious?
Toxicology tests (tox screens) are performed to screen for the use of medication (toxin) and for the underlying cause of the patient's unusual behavior and the reason the patient is unconscious.

2.16 Why would the folic acid test be administered to a pregnant woman?

The folic acid test is performed to screen for malnutrition, anemia, and malabsorption, and assess the treatment of folic acid deficiency and the level of folic acid during pregnancy to reduce the risk of birth defects.

2.17 Why would the gastrin test be ordered?

The gastrin test is performed to screen for Zollinger-Ellison syndrome, pernicious anemia, pancreatic tumors, and G-cell hyperplasia.

2.18 What is the function of the ferritin test?

The ferritin test is performed to screen for hemochromatosis (excess iron), iron deficiency anemia, inflammation, and assess for the treatment of hemochromatosis and iron deficiency anemia.

2.19 Why would the health care provider order the lactic acid test?

The lactic acid test is performed to screen for lactic acidosis, tissue oxygenation, and the underlying cause of acidosis.

2.20 What test would the health care provider order to assess the therapeutic level of warfarin?

The health care provider would order the prothrombin time (PT) test to assess the therapeutic level of warfarin.

2.21 Why is the reticulocyte count test ordered?

The test is performed to screen for anemia and assess the treatment of anemia.

2.22 What is the purpose of the Schilling test?

The Schilling test is performed to assess the absorption of vitamin B_{12} and the production of the intrinsic factor.

2.23 Why would the sedimentation rate (SED) test be ordered?

The test is performed to screen for inflammation and to assess treatment for inflammation.

2.24 What test might be ordered to assess the treatment for iron deficiency anemia?

The iron (Fe) test might be ordered to assess the treatment for iron deficiency anemia.

2.25 What is the goal of the serum protein electrophoresis (SPE) test?

The test is performed to screen for amyloidosis, multiple myeloma, and macroglobulinemia, and assess the underlying cause of hypogammaglobulinemia.

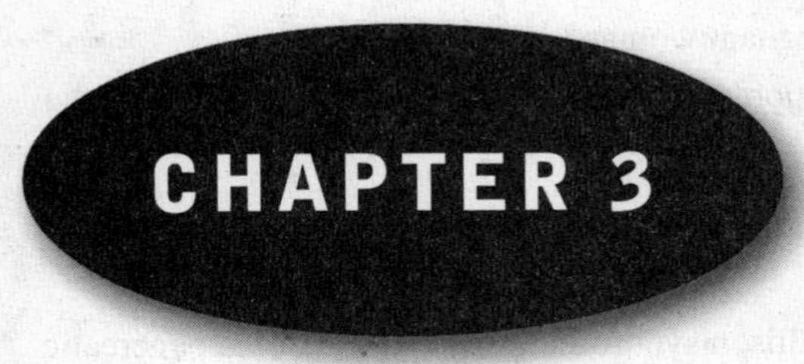

Electrolyte Tests

3.1 Definition

Electrolytes are salts that are electrically charged ions used to maintain voltage across cell membranes and carry electrical impulses within the body. The concentration of electrolytes within the body is constantly changing. The kidney is the main regulatory organ that adjusts electrolyte levels to maintain a balance. Electrolyte tests are referred to as electrolyte, basic metabolic, or comprehensive metabolic panel. An electrolyte panel measures only electrolytes in a sample of blood. The basic metabolic and comprehensive metabolic panels measure electrolytes and other components.

3.2 Calcium (Ca) Test

The calcium (Ca) electrolyte test is used to screen for parathyroid gland function, kidney function, kidney stones, pancreatitis, and bone disease. The test also assesses the underlying cause of muscle spasms, depression, confusion, tingling around the mouth and fingers, muscle cramping, and twitching that are caused by low calcium levels in the blood; nausea, vomiting, bone pain, lack of appetite, weakness, abdominal pain, constipation, and increased urination that are caused by a high calcium level in the blood; and abnormal electrocardiogram.

Understanding the Calcium Test

Calcium is required for growth of bones and teeth and for muscle contraction and blood clotting. Nearly all calcium in the body is stored in bone with a minimum amount in blood. Calcium has a homeostatic relationship with phosphate. Calcium increases in blood as phosphate decreases, and calcium decreases when phosphate increases in the blood.

The parathyroid keeps calcium and phosphate balanced. Where there is too much phosphate (too little calcium) in blood, the parathyroid releases the parathyroid hormone (PTH) that stimulates osteoclast, breaking down bone to increase the calcium level in blood. PTH also activates vitamin D to increase absorption of calcium in the gastrointestinal tract. Vitamin D is necessary for calcium absorption and for the kidneys to retain calcium. Too much calcium in the blood causes the thyroid gland to release calcitonin, which moves calcium from blood to bone.

There are two kinds of calcium blood tests that are performed as part of a routine blood screening. The *nonionized calcium test* measures calcium attached to albumin in the blood. This test is affected by the amount of albumin in the blood. The *ionized calcium test* measures calcium not attached to albumin in the blood, and therefore is not affected by the amount of albumin in the blood.

3.3 Magnesium (Mg) Test

The magnesium (Mg) test is used to assess the effects of medication that cause changes in the level of magnesium and for the therapeutic treatment of high and low levels of magnesium. The test is also used to assess the underlying cause of muscle weakness, muscle twitches, muscle irritability, arrhythmia, nausea, vomiting, low blood pressure, and dizziness.

Understanding the Magnesium Test

Magnesium, found mostly in bones and inside cells, is an electrolyte used to transfer potassium and sodium in and out of cells and is used to activate nerves, muscles, and enzymes. The magnesium blood test measures the level of magnesium in a blood sample and is tested along with other electrolytes.

3.4 Phosphate Test

The phosphate test is used to screen for kidney and bone disease, and to assess parathyroid gland function.

Understanding the Phosphate Test

Phosphorus is a mineral that contains a particle called phosphate, which is necessary for growth of bones and teeth, and for contracting muscles. Most phosphate is in bone. Phosphate and calcium have an inverse relationship. The phosphate test measures the level of phosphate in the blood.

3.5 Potassium (K) Test

The potassium (K) test is used to screen for cell lysis syndrome, and to assess the effect of total parenteral nutrition (TPN), the adverse effects of diuretics, the effects of kidney dialysis, and the underlying cause of high blood pressure.

Understanding the Potassium Test

Potassium is a mineral stored inside the cell that has multiple functions, including muscle contractions, neural transmission, and fluid balance. Potassium is excreted by the kidneys and regulated by the hormone aldosterone released by the adrenal glands. Potassium and sodium have an inverse relationship. The potassium test measures the level of potassium in blood.

3.6 Sodium (Na) Test

The sodium (Na) test is used to screen for adrenal gland disease, electrolyte balance, water balance, and kidney disease.

Understanding the Sodium Test

Sodium is a mineral stored outside the cell in blood and lymph fluid that has multiple functions, including muscle contractions, neural transmission, and fluid balance. Sodium is excreted by the kidneys, regulated by the hormone aldosterone, and released by the adrenal glands. Sodium and potassium have an inverse relationship. The sodium test measures the level of sodium in blood.

3.7 Chloride (Cl) Test

The chloride (Cl) test is administered to assess the underlying cause of metabolic alkalosis, kidney disorder, adrenal gland disorder, confusion, muscle spasms, muscle weakness, and difficulty breathing.

Understanding the Chloride Test

Chloride is an electrolyte found outside the cell and is involved in fluid balance. The chloride test measures the level of chloride in blood.

Solved Problems

Electrolyte Tests

3.1 What are electrolytes?

Electrolytes are salts that are electrically charged ions used to maintain voltage across cell membranes and carry electrical impulses within the body.

3.2 What organ adjusts electrolytes?

The kidney makes adjustments to keep electrolytes in balance.

3.3 What are other names for electrolyte tests?

Electrolyte tests are referred to as electrolyte, basic metabolic, or comprehensive metabolic panels.

3.4 What is measured by an electrolyte panel?

An electrolyte panel measures only electrolytes in a sample of blood.

3.5 What is measured by a basic metabolic panel and a comprehensive metabolic panel?

The basic metabolic and comprehensive metabolic panels measure electrolytes and other components.

3.6 Why would the calcium test be ordered?

The calcium electrolyte test is used to screen for parathyroid gland function, kidney function, kidney stones, pancreatitis, and bone disease. The test also assesses the underlying cause of muscle spasms, depression, confusion, tingling around the mouth and fingers, muscle cramping, and twitching that are caused by low calcium levels in the blood; nausea, vomiting, bone pain, lack of appetite, weakness, abdominal pain, constipation, and increased urination that are caused by a high calcium level in the blood; and abnormal electrocardiogram.

3.7 Calcium has a homeostatic relationship with what other electrolyte?

Calcium has a homeostatic relationship with phosphate.

3.8 What keeps calcium and phosphate in balance?

Parathyroid keeps calcium and phosphate in balance.

3.9 What removes calcium from blood to bone?

Too much calcium in the blood causes the thyroid gland to release calcitonin, which moves calcium from blood to bone.

3.10 What is the ionized calcium test?

The ionized calcium test measures calcium not attached to albumin in the blood and therefore is not affected by the amount of albumin in the blood.

3.11 What is the nonionized calcium test?

The nonionized calcium test measures calcium attached to albumin in the blood. This test is affected by the amount of albumin in the blood.

3.12 Why might the health care provider order a magnesium test?

The magnesium test is used to assess the effects of medication that causes changes in the level of magnesium and helps determine the therapeutic treatment of high and low levels of magnesium. The test is also used to assess the underlying cause of muscle weakness, muscle twitches, muscle irritability, arrhythmia, nausea, vomiting, low blood pressure, and dizziness.

3.13 What is the function of magnesium?

Magnesium, found mostly in bones and inside cells, is an electrolyte and is used to transfer potassium and sodium in and out of cells. It is used to activate nerves, muscles, and enzymes.

3.14 What is the purpose of administering the phosphate test?

The test is used to screen for kidney and bone disease, and to assess parathyroid gland function.

3.15 What is the function of phosphate?

Phosphate is necessary for growth of bones and teeth and for contracting muscles.

3.16 What is the difference between phosphate and phosphorus?

Phosphorus is a mineral that contains a particle called phosphate.

3.17 Why is the potassium test ordered?

The potassium test is used to screen for cell lysis syndrome and assess the effect of total parenteral nutrition (TPN) and kidney dialysis, the adverse effect of diuretics, and to assess the underlying cause of high blood pressure.

3.18 Where is potassium stored in the body?

Potassium is a mineral stored inside the cell.

3.19 What is the function of potassium?

Potassium has multiple functions including muscle contractions, neural transmission, and fluid balance.

3.20 What regulates potassium?

Potassium is regulated by the hormone aldosterone released by the adrenal glands.

3.21 By what organ is potassium excreted?

Potassium is excreted by the kidneys.

3.22 What electrolyte has an inverse relationship with potassium?

Potassium and sodium have an inverse relationship.

3.23 Why is the sodium test ordered?

The sodium test is used to screen for adrenal gland disease, electrolyte balance, water balance, and kidney disease.

3.24 Where is sodium located in the body?

Sodium is a mineral stored outside the cell in blood and lymph fluid.

3.25 What is the function of sodium in the body?

Sodium has multiple functions including muscle contractions, neural transmission, and fluid balance.

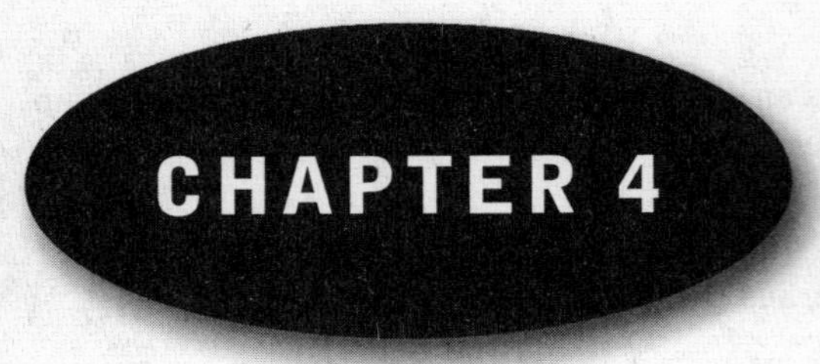

Liver Tests

4.1 Definition

The liver is the largest gland in the body that produces and secretes substances. The liver synthesizes albumin, which maintains blood volume and clotting factors. The liver also synthesizes, stores, and metabolizes fatty acids and cholesterol. Fatty acids are used for energy by the body. The liver stores and metabolizes carbohydrates. Carbohydrates are converted into glucose for energy.

The liver forms and secretes bile. Bile contains acids that help the intestines absorb fats and vitamins A, D, E, and K, which are fat-soluble vitamins. In addition, the liver clears the body of medications and harmful chemicals such as bilirubin, which is the result of the metabolism of aged red blood cells, and ammonia, which is the result of metabolism of proteins. The liver transforms these chemicals into components that are easily excreted by the body in urine or stool.

4.2 Hepatitis A Virus (HAV) Test

The hepatitis A virus (HAV) test is performed to screen for hepatitis A virus infection and the effectiveness of the hepatitis A vaccine.

Understanding the Hepatitis A Virus Test

A patient who is or has been infected with the hepatitis A virus (HAV) will have hepatitis A antibodies in his or her blood. A patient who received the hepatitis A vaccine will also have these antibodies, indicating the effectiveness of the vaccine. If not recently immunized, these antibodies indicate pathology versus adequate titers from being immunized. There are two types of antibodies:

- **IgM anti-HAV:** The presence of this antibody indicates that the patient was recently infected. This antibody is detectable 2 weeks after being infected and remains in the blood for 3 to 12 months.
- **IgG anti-HAV:** The presence of this antibody indicates that the patient has been infected at some point. This antibody is detectable 8 to 12 weeks following the infection and remains in the blood.

4.3 Hepatitis B Virus (HBV) Test

Hepatitis B virus (HBV) tests are performed to screen for hepatitis B virus infection and the effectiveness of the hepatitis B vaccine and treatment for a hepatitis B virus infection. These tests are also used to assess if blood designated for transfusion is infected with the hepatitis B virus.

Understanding the Hepatitis B Virus Tests

Hepatitis B is a virus that can cause an infection. There are several hepatitis B virus tests used to determine if blood has signs of HBV. There are three signs:

- **HBV antibodies:** HBV antibodies are produced as part of the immune response to the presence of HBV in the patient and may remain in the patient's blood long after HBV is destroyed.
- **HBV antigens:** HBV antigens are markers created by HBV when HBV infects the patient.
- **HBV DNA:** HBV DNA is present when HBV infects the patient.

There are seven types of HBV tests:

1. **Hepatitis B Surface Antigen (HBsAg):** This is the first test that detects HBV antigen even before symptoms are present. It is also used to detect if the patient will be an HBV carrier if the HBsAg level is elevated >6 months.
2. **Hepatitis B Surface Antibody (HBsAb):** This test detects HBV antibodies, which are elevated 4 weeks after HBsAg is no longer detectable. The test is used to determine if the patient requires an HBV vaccination.
3. **Hepatitis B e-Antigen (HBeAg):** This test detects the HBeAg antigen that is present if the patient is currently infected and is used to monitor HBV treatment.
4. **Hepatitis DNA Test:** This test determines the level of HBV DNA in the patient's blood and is used to monitor treatment for chronic HBV infection.
5. **Hepatitis B Core Antibody (HBcAb):** This test detects the HBcAb antibody a month after the HBV infection and is used to screen transfused blood for hepatitis B.
6. **Hepatitis B Core Antibody IgM (HBcAbIgM):** This test detects the HBcAbIgM antibody within 6 months of the patient becoming infected with HBV.
7. **Hepatitis B e-Antibody (HBeAb):** This test detects the HBeAb antibody, indicating that the patient has almost recovered from an acute HBV infection.

4.4 Alanine Aminotransferase (ALT) Test

The alanine aminotransferase (ALT) test is performed to screen for liver disorder and assess the underlying cause of jaundice. This test is also administered to assess for side effects of medications that can cause liver damage.

Understanding the Alanine Aminotransferase Test

Alanine aminotransferase, formerly called serum glutamic pyruvic transaminase (SGPT), is an enzyme mainly found in the liver, but is also in the heart, pancreas, muscles, and kidneys in small amounts. Damage to the liver caused by injury or disease results in the release of ALT in the blood. The ALT test measures the level of ALT in the blood as a way to detect liver disease.

4.5 Alkaline Phosphatase (ALP) Test

The alkaline phosphatase (ALP) test is used to screen for liver disorder and to assess the side effects of medications that can cause liver damage. This test is also used to screen for rickets, osteomalacia, Paget's disease and bone tumor, along with assessing the effectiveness of treatment of these diseases. It is also administered to assess the underlying cause of high calcium level in blood.

Understanding the Alkaline Phosphatase Test

Alkaline phosphatase is an enzyme produced mainly in the liver and is also produced by bones, kidneys, intestines, and placenta. The ALP test measures the level of ALP in blood.

An alkaline phosphatase isoenzymes test is likely to be ordered if the ALP level is high. The health care provider may order an ultrasound or CT scan. The gamma glutamyl transferase (GGT), 5-nucleotidase, or the gamma glutamyl transpeptidase (GGTP) test might be ordered if the ALP level is high to differentiate between bone ALP and liver ALP.

4.6 Ammonia Test

The ammonia test is performed to screen for liver disorder and assess the treatment of liver disease. It is also administered to screen for Reye's syndrome, hyperalimentation, cirrhosis, and acute liver failure.

Understanding the Amonia Test

Ammonia is formed when bacteria in the intestines break down protein. Ammonia is then converted into urea by the liver, which is excreted by the kidney in urine. The ammonia test measures the ammonia level in the blood. If the liver is unable to convert ammonia to urea, ammonia levels in blood increase, indicating that there may be a liver function problem.

4.7 Aspartate Aminotransferase (AST) Test

The aspartate aminotransferase (AST) test is used to screen for liver disorder, hepatitis, and cirrhosis. It is also administered to assess treatment of liver disease, side effects of medication that cause liver damage, and the underlying cause of jaundice.

Understanding the Aspartate Aminotransferase Test

Aspartate aminotransferase, previously known as serum glutamic oxaloacetic transaminase (SGOT), is an enzyme in the liver, heart, pancreas, kidneys, red blood cells, and muscle tissues. When these tissues or cells are damaged there is an increase of AST in the blood 6 to 10 hours after the damage that remains for 4 days. The AST test measures the level of AST in the blood.

The health care provider orders tests to measure AST and ALT in a normal screen for liver damage and liver disease. The AST test is more effective in detecting liver damage caused by alcohol abuse than the ALT test. As the patient recovers from tissue damage, the AST level in the blood decreases.

4.8 Bilirubin Test

The bilirubin test is used to screen for liver disorder, hepatitis, cirrhosis, blocked bile duct from gallstone or pancreatic tumor, hemolytic anemia, hemolytic disease, neonatal jaundice, and the side effect of medication that causes liver damage.

Understanding the Bilirubin Test

The liver breaks down old red blood cells into bilirubin, which becomes the brownish yellow component of bile. Bilirubin is excreted through feces. Bilirubin gives feces its brown color. Indirect (unconjugated) bilirubin, which is insoluble in water, is carried by the blood to the liver, where indirect bilirubin is transformed into direct bilirubin, which is soluble in water. The bilirubin test measures the total bilirubin level in the blood and the direct bilirubin level in the blood. Indirect bilirubin is measured by subtracting the direct bilirubin level from the total bilirubin level.

Solved Problems

Liver Tests

4.1 What does the liver synthesize, store, and metabolize?

The liver synthesizes, stores, and metabolizes fatty acids and cholesterol.

4.2 What does the liver form and secrete?

The liver forms and secretes bile.

4.3 How does the liver clear the body of medication and harmful chemicals?

The liver transforms these chemicals into components that are easily excreted by the body in urine or stool.

4.4 What is the purpose of the hepatitis A virus (HAV) test?

The HAV test is used to screen for hepatitis A virus infection and the effectiveness of the hepatitis A vaccine.

4.5 What is IgM anti-HAV?

The presence of the antibody IgM anti-HAV indicates that the patient was recently infected. This antibody is detectable 2 weeks after being infected and remains in the blood for 3 to 12 months.

4.6 What are hepatitis B virus (HBV) antigens?

HBV antigens are markers created by the HBV when HBV infects the patient.

4.7 What are HBV antibodies?

HBV antibodies are produced as part of the immune response to the presence of HBV in the patient and may remain in the patient's blood long after HBV is destroyed.

4.8 What is the hepatitis B surface antigen (HBsAg) test?

HBsAg is the first test that detects HBV antigen even before symptoms are present. It is also used to detect if the patient will be an HBV carrier, if the HBsAg level is elevated >6 months.

4.9 What is the hepatitis B e-antigen (HBeAg) test?

HBeAg detects the HBeAg antigen, which is present if the patient is currently infected and is used to monitor HBV treatment.

4.10 What is the hepatitis B core antibody (HBcAb) test?

HBcAb detects the HBcAb antibody a month after the HBV infection and is used to screen transfused blood for hepatitis B.

4.11 What is the hepatitis B e-antibody (HBeAB) test?

The HBeAb test detects the HBeAb antibody, indicating that the patient has almost recovered from an acute HBV infection.

4.12 What is the purpose of the alanine aminotransferase (ALT)test?

The ALT test is used to screen for liver disorder and assess the underlying cause of jaundice. This test is also administered to assess the side effects of medications that can cause liver damage.

4.13 What is alanine aminotransferase?

Alanine aminotransferase, formerly called serum glutamic pyruvic transaminase (SGPT), is an enzyme mainly found in the liver; but it is also present in the heart, pancreas, muscles, and kidneys in small amounts.

4.14 Why is alanine aminotransferase measured in the blood?

Damage to the liver caused by injury or disease results in the release of ALT in the blood.

4.15 What is the purpose of the alkaline phosphatase (ALP) test?

The ALP test is used to screen for liver disorder and assess the side effects of medications that can cause liver damage. This test is also used to screen for rickets, osteomalacia, Paget's disease, and bone tumor, along with assessing the effectiveness of treatment of these diseases. It is also administered to assess the underlying cause of high calcium levels in the blood.

4.16 Why is the ammonia test ordered?

The ammonia test is performed to screen for liver disorder and assess the treatment of liver disease. It is also administered to screen for Reye's syndrome, hyperalimentation, cirrhosis, and acute liver failure.

4.17 How is ammonia formed?

Ammonia is formed when bacteria in the intestines break down protein.

4.18 What is the relationship between ammonia and the liver?

Ammonia is then converted into urea by the liver, which is excreted by the kidney in urine.

4.19 Why is ammonia measured in blood?

If the liver is unable to convert ammonia to urea, ammonia levels in blood increase, indicating that there may be a liver function problem.

4.20 What is aspartate aminotransferase (AST)?

AST, previously known as serum glutamic oxaloacetic transaminase (SGOT), is an enzyme in the liver, heart, pancreas, kidneys, red blood cells, and muscle tissues.

4.21 How long will AST remain in the blood?

When the liver, heart, pancreas, kidneys, red blood cells, and muscle tissues or cells are damaged, there is an increase of AST in the blood 6 to 10 hours after the damage and it remains for 4 days.

4.22 What is bilirubin?

The liver breaks down old red blood cells into bilirubin, which becomes the brownish yellow component of bile.

4.23 What is indirect bilirubin?

Indirect bilirubin is carried by the blood to the liver where indirect bilirubin is transformed into direct bilirubin.

4.24 What is the difference between direct and indirect bilirubin?

Indirect (unconjugated) bilirubin is insoluble in water. Direct bilirubin is soluble in water.

4.25 What is the relationship between feces and bilirubin?

Bilirubin gives feces its brown color.

Cardiac Enzymes and Markers Tests

5.1 Definition

Cardiac muscle contains enzymes. In a myocardial infarction (MI) (heart attack), cardiac muscle is damaged, causing the release of cardiac enzymes into the bloodstream. When a patient is suspected of having a MI, the health care provider will order cardiac enzymes and cardiac marker tests to determine if cardiac muscle enzymes appear in the patient's blood.

It can take 2 to 24 hours for cardiac muscle enzymes to reach a detectable level in blood. Therefore, health care providers typically use an electrocardiogram (EKG or ECG) to diagnose the acute phase of a MI. The cardiac enzymes and cardiac markers tests are used to confirm a previous acute MI.

There are several cardiac enzymes and cardiac marker tests commonly used by health care providers to confirm a myocardial infarction diagnosis.

5.2 Brain Natriuretic Peptide (BNP) Test

The brain natriuretic peptide (BNP) test is used to screen for heart failure and assess treatment for heart failure.

Understanding the Brain Natriuretic Peptide Test

The heart produces the hormone brain natriuretic peptide. A low level of BNP is normally found in blood. However, the BNP level increases when the heart works harder for long periods, such as in heart failure. The BNP test measures the level of BNP in the blood.

The health care provider may order the N-terminal probrain natriuretic peptide (NT-proBNP) test that measures the NT-proBNP hormone. This test provides diagnostic results that are similar to the BNP test.

5.3 Cardiac Enzyme Studies

Cardiac enzyme studies screen for an MI, cardiac muscle injury following bypass surgery, and unstable angina. It is also used to assess the results of percutaneous coronary intervention (PCI) or thrombolytic medication to restore blood flow through the coronary artery.

Understanding Cardiac Enzyme Studies

The cells of heart muscles and other tissues contain the enzyme creatinine phosphokinase (CPK) and the protein troponin (TnT, TnI). Creatinine phosphokinase and troponin enter the blood when heart muscle and other tissues are damaged. If levels of CPK and troponin are high, the health care provider orders an EKG to differentiate between heart muscle damage and other tissue damage. Troponin and CPK-MB are mostly found in cardiac muscle.

Blood samples are taken every 12 hours for 2 days following a suspected heart attack. It takes 6 hours for troponin levels to rise after a heart attack. The health care provider may order a myoglobin (MB) test along with the cardiac enzymes test to help diagnose a heart attack.

5.4 Homocysteine Test

The homocysteine test is used to assess risk for stroke and a heart attack.

Understanding the Homocysteine Test

Homocysteine is an amino acid found in blood, and the homocysteine test measures the level of homocysteine in blood. Homocysteine levels increase along with increased levels of cholesterol, which can lead to a risk of stroke, deep venous thrombosis, heart attack, and pulmonary embolism. The health care provider may order the homocysteine test for a patient who has a family history of heart disease but has not exhibited other risk factors. The health care provider may order a urine homocysteine test.

5.5 Renin Assay Test

The renin assay test is used to assess the underlying cause of hypertension.

Understanding the Renin Assay Test

Blood pressure is regulated by the renin angiotensin system (RAS). Low blood pressure causes the secretion of the renin enzyme by the kidneys, which increases angiotensin production. This increase constricts blood vessels, resulting in increased blood pressure. Angiotensin causes the adrenal cortex to replace aldosterone, causing the kidneys to retain water and sodium, which results in an increase in fluid volume and blood pressure. The renin assay test measures the level of renin in blood.

The health care provider may also order the aldosterone test. The renin stimulation test may be ordered if the renin level is low.

Solved Problems

Cardiac Enzymes and Markers Test

5.1 How long can it take before cardiac enzymes reach a detectable level in blood?

It can take 2 to 24 hours for cardiac muscle enzymes to reach a detectable level in blood.

5.2 What test is administered in the acute phase of a myocardial infarction (MI)?

Health care providers typically use an EKG to diagnose the acute phase of a MI.

5.3 What test might be ordered if the renin level is low?

The renin stimulation test.

5.4 What is the purpose of the brain natriuretic peptide (BNP) test?

The BNP test is used to screen for heart failure and assess the correct treatment.

5.5 What is BNP?

The heart produces the hormone brain natriuretic peptide.

5.6 Why is BNP measured?

The BNP level increases when the heart works harder for long periods, such as in heart failure.

5.7 What other hormone test might the health care provider order in addition to the BNP test?

The health care provider may order the N-terminal probrain natriuretic peptide (NT-proBNP) test, which measures the NT-proBNP hormone. This test provides diagnostic results similar to the BNP test.

5.8 What test might be administered following percutaneous coronary intervention (PCI) or thrombolytic medication to restore blood flow through the coronary artery?

Cardiac enzyme studies might be administered to restore blood flow through the coronary artery.

5.9 What test is administered following bypass surgery and why is it administered?

The cardiac enzyme studies test is administered to assess cardiac muscle injury following bypass surgery.

5.10 What is measured in the cardiac enzyme studies test?

Creatinine phosphokinase (CPK) and the protein troponin (TnT, TnI) are measured in the cardiac enzyme studies test.

5.11 Why might the health care provider order an EKG if CPK and troponin are high?

The health care provider might order an electrocardiogram to differentiate between heart muscle damage and other tissue damage.

5.12 Which enzyme and protein are mostly found in cardiac muscle?

Troponin and CPK-MB are mostly found in cardiac muscle.

5.13 How long does it take troponin levels to rise in blood following a myocardial infarction?

It takes 6 hours for troponin levels to rise after a heart attack.

5.14 How many times is the cardiac enzyme studies test administered following a suspected heart attack?

Blood samples are taken every 12 hours for 2 days following a suspected heart attack.

5.15 What is homocysteine?

Homocysteine is an amino acid found in blood.

5.16 What is the purpose of the homocysteine test?

The homocysteine test is used to assess risk for stroke and heart attack.

5.17 Why might a health care provider order the homocysteine test?

The health care provider may order the homocysteine test for a patient who has a family history of heart disease but has not exhibited other risk factors.

5.18 Why is homocysteine measured?

Homocysteine is measured because increased homocysteine levels along with increased levels of cholesterol can lead to a risk of stroke, deep venous thrombosis, heart attack, and pulmonary embolism.

5.19 Where is homocysteine measured?

Homocysteine is measured in blood and urine.

5.20 What is the purpose of the renin assay test?

The renin assay test is used to assess the underlying cause of hypertension.

5.21 How is blood pressure regulated?

Blood pressure is regulated by the renin angiotensin system (RAS).

5.22 What occurs during low blood pressure?

Low blood pressure causes the secretion of the renin enzyme by the kidneys, which increases angiotensin production and constricts blood vessels, resulting in increased blood pressure.

5.23 What is the function of angiotensin?

Angiotensin causes the adrenal cortex to replace aldosterone, causing the kidneys to retain water and sodium, and resulting in an increase in fluid volume and blood pressure.

5.24 What does the renin assay test measure?

The renin assay test measures the level of renin in the blood.

5.25 What would a high level of renin in blood indicate?

A high level of renin in the blood would indicate high blood pressure.

Serology Tests

6.1 Definition

The presence of foreign protein in the body from a microorganism or mismatched donated blood causes a reaction of the body's immune system. This reaction produces antibodies that destroy the foreign protein by metabolizing it into components that can be excreted safely by the body.

Serology tests examine the patient's blood serum for antibodies. Health care providers order serology tests for a number of purposes. These include diagnosing an infection, determining if the patient has developed immunity to specific antigens, determining a patient's blood type, and determining if the patient has an autoimmune disorder.

An autoimmune disorder occurs when the patient's immune system identifies the patient's own protein as a foreign protein, resulting in the patient's immune system creating antibodies to that protein.

6.2 Immunoglobulin (Ig) Tests

Immunoglobulin tests are used to screen for allergies, autoimmune disease, multiple myeloma, and macroglobulinemia cancer. They are also used to assess the strength of the immune system, the patient's immunization, and the effectiveness of treatment for infection and bone marrow cancer. An immunoglobulin test is commonly administered as a follow-up to an abnormal result from the total blood protein or blood protein electrophoresis test.

Understanding Immunoglobulin Tests

Immunoglobulins are antibodies made by the immune system in response to microorganisms that enter the body, allergens, and abnormal cells such as cancer cells. An antibody is specific to an antigen. The immunoglobulin tests measure the level of an immunoglobulin in the patient's blood. A low level of a specific immunoglobulin increases the risk of repeated infections from an antigen. There are five major types of immunoglobulins:

1. **IgA:** This is found in tears and saliva and protects the ears, eyes, breathing passages, digestive tract, and vagina, which are exposed to outside antigens. It comprises 10% of immunoglobulins.
2. **IgG:** This is found in all body fluids and defends the body against viruses and bacteria. This immunoglobulin crosses the placenta. It comprises 80% of immunoglobulins.
3. **IgM:** This is found in blood and lymph fluid and is the first response to infection. It comprises 5% of immunoglobulins, and forms when an infection occurs for the first time.
4. **IgE:** This is found in mucous membranes, lungs, and skin and defends against allergens. A high level of IgE immunoglobulin is common in patients who are hypoallergenic. It comprises <5% of immunoglobulins.
5. **IgD:** This is found in abdominal and chest tissues. It comprises <5% of immunoglobulins.

6.3 Antinuclear Antibodies (ANA) Test

The antinuclear antibodies (ANA) test is used to screen for rheumatoid arthritis, systemic lupus erythematosus (SLE), polymyositis, and scleroderma.

Understanding the Antinuclear Antibodies Test

In autoimmune diseases, the body produces antibodies that attach and destroy the body's own cells. The antinuclear antibody test measures the pattern and amount of these antibodies.

6.4 Human Immunodeficiency Virus (HIV) Tests

Human immunodeficiency virus (HIV) tests are used to assess if the patient has been infected with HIV.

Understanding Human Immunodeficiency Virus Tests

The human immunodeficiency virus infects the CD4+ white blood cells that are the body's defense against infection. There are two types of HIV. *HIV-1* is common in nearly all acquired immunodeficiency syndrome (AIDS) cases. *HIV-2* is associated with West Africa. HIV causes AIDS, which is incurable. There is a period when the HIV infection is not detectable in a patient. This is called the *seroconversion period,* also known as the *window period.* The patient can spread HIV during this period. The seroconversion period can be up to 2 weeks and as long as 6 months. After the seroconversion period, the HIV test is able to detect HIV antibodies or the HIV's RNA in the patient's blood.

There are several HIV tests:

- **Enzyme-Linked Immunosorbent Assay (ELISA):** The first test administered to screen a patient. This looks for HIV antibodies in the blood. If the test result is negative, then other tests are not performed. If the test result is positive, another ELISA test is performed. Other tests are performed if there are two positive ELISA tests because the ELISA test can produce a false-positive result.
- **Western Blot:** This tests for HIV antibodies and is more difficult to perform than the ELISA test.
- **Polymerase Chain Reaction (PCR):** This looks for HIV's RNA in the blood. Polymerase chain reaction is used to identify a very recent infection and is administered to screen blood and organs before donations and when HIV antibody tests are inconclusive. The PCR test is not performed often because of expense.
- **Indirect Fluorescent Antibody (IFA):** This tests for HIV antibodies and is performed secondary to two positive ELISA tests.
- **Saliva Test:** Tests the presence of HIV in saliva. Results must be confirmed by the Western blot test.
- **Rapid Test Kits:** Test results are available in a half hour. Results must be confirmed by the Western blot test.
- **Home Blood Test Kits:** This is available without prescription. Samples are sent through the mail to the laboratory. Results are provided over the phone using an anonymous code.

Detecting HIV in a newborn is difficult because the newborn's blood still has HIV antibodies from either HIV-positive parent for 18 months.

Testing is performed when the patient:

- Exhibits symptoms of HIV
- Has HIV risk factors
- Is donating blood or organs
- Is pregnant. An infected mother can be treated, decreasing the likelihood that HIV will be passed to the fetus

6.5 CD4+ Count Test

The CD4+ count is used to assess the patient's immune system, as well as the progress and treatment of HIV; assist in the diagnosis of AIDS; and develop a baseline CD4+ count. The baseline is then compared with values over time to identify changes in levels.

Understanding the CD4+ Count Test

Three types of leukocytes (white blood cells, WBCs) important to fighting infection are *T lymphocytes, T cells,* and *T-helper cells*. The CD4+ count test measures the level of these leukocytes to assess the patient's immune system. Patients who have a low CD4+ count are at risk for opportunistic infections.

The CD4+ count test is used to assess the immune system of patients who have HIV. The result of the CD4+ count test and the viral load test determines when antiretroviral treatment for HIV is started. The health care provider may also order the CD4+ percentage test that determines the percentage of CD4+ cells in the total number of lymphocytes and the CD8 count test that determines the level of T-suppressor cells.

6.6 Viral Load Measurement Test

The viral load measurement test is used to assess the progress and treatment of HIV infection.

Understanding the Viral Load Measurement Test

HIV in a patient's blood is determined by the presence of HIV RNA. The amount of HIV RNA indicates if the infection is decreasing, stabilized, or increasing. The viral load measurement test determines the amount of HIV RNA in the patient's blood. A viral load measurement test is administered when the patient is diagnosed with HIV and becomes the baseline. Results of subsequent viral load measurement tests are compared with the baseline to determine the infection's progress.

There are three types of viral load measurement tests:

1. Branched DNA (bDNA) test
2. Nucleic acid sequence-based amplification (NASBA) test
3. Reverse-transcriptase polymerase chain reaction (RT-PCR) test

The health care provider may order the CD4+ count test along with the viral load measurement test, although the viral load measurement test is more accurate than the CD4+ count test to assess the progress of the HIV infection. The viral load measurement test is not used to diagnose HIV.

A patient diagnosed with HIV who has a negative viral load measurement test result can infect another person.

6.7 Rheumatoid Factor (RF) Test

The rheumatoid factor (RF) test is used to screen for rheumatoid arthritis.

Understanding the Rheumatoid Factor Test

The RF is an autoantibody that destroys the patient's own tissues, resulting in stiffness, joint pain, and inflammation. The RF test measures the amount of the RF in the blood sample and is used to differentiate rheumatoid arthritis from other forms of arthritis. There are two types of RF tests—the agglutination test and the nephelometry test.

The RF is one of other signs and symptoms used to diagnose rheumatoid arthritis. A patient may have a high level of RF but no symptoms of rheumatoid arthritis. However, the patient is likely to develop rheumatoid arthritis in the future. A patient who has a normal level of RF and symptoms of rheumatoid arthritis will likely require a second RF test.

Solved Problems

Serology Tests

6.1 What is the purpose of serology tests?

Serology tests examine the patient's blood serum for antibodies.

6.2 What is an antibody?

The presence of foreign protein in the body from a microorganism or mismatched donated blood causes a reaction of the body's immune system. This reaction produces antibodies that destroy the foreign protein by metabolizing it into components that can be excreted safely by the body.

6.3 What is an autoimmune disorder?

An autoimmune disorder occurs when the patient's immune system identifies the patient's own protein as a foreign protein, resulting in the patient's immune system creating antibodies to that protein.

6.4 What is the purpose of the immunoglobulin tests?

Immunoglobulin tests are used to screen for allergies, autoimmune disease, multiple myeloma, and macroglobulinemia cancer. They are also used to assess the strength of the immune system, the patient's immunization, and the effectiveness of treatment for infection and bone marrow cancer.

6.5 What are immunoglobulins?

Immunoglobulins are antibodies made by the immune system in response to microorganisms that enter the body, allergens, and abnormal cells such as cancer cells.

6.6 What is the risk of having a low level of a specific immunoglobulin?

A low level of a specific immunoglobulin increases the risk of repeated infections from an antigen.

6.7 What is IgA?

IgA is an immunoglobulin found in tears and saliva that protects the ears, eyes, breathing passages, digestive tract, and vagina, which are exposed to outside antigens.

6.8 What immunoglobulin defends the body against viruses and bacteria?

IgG is found in all body fluids and defends the body against viruses and bacteria.

6.9 What immunoglobulin is the first response to infection?

IgM is found in blood and lymph fluid and is the first response to infection. It forms when an infection occurs for the first time.

6.10 What immunoglobulin defends against allergens?

IgE is found in mucous membranes, lungs, and skin and defends against allergens. A high level of IgE immunoglobulin is common in patients who are hyperallergenic.

6.11 What immunoglobulin crosses the placenta?

IgG crosses the placenta.

6.12 What is the purpose of the antinuclear antibodies (ANA) test?

The ANA test is used to screen for rheumatoid arthritis, systemic lupus erythematosus (SLE), polymyositis, and scleroderma.

6.13 What does the ANA test measure?

It measures antibodies that attach and destroy the body's own cells.

6.14 What does the human immunodeficiency virus (HIV) infect?

The HIV infects the CD4+ white blood cells that are the body's defense against infection.

6.15 During what period is the HIV test ineffective?

There is a period when the HIV infection is not detectable in a patient. This is called the seroconversion period, also known as the window period. The patient can spread HIV during this period. The seroconversion period can be up to 2 weeks and as long as 6 months.

6.16 What is enzyme-linked immunosorbent assay (ELISA) test?

The ELISA is the first test administered to screen a patient. It looks for HIV antibodies in the blood.

6.17 What is the polymerase chain reaction (PCR) test?

The PCR test looks for HIV's RNA in the blood. PCR is used to identify a very recent infection and is administered to screen blood and organs before donations and when HIV antibody tests are inconclusive.

6.18 Why is the PCR test not performed frequently?

The PCR test is not performed often because of expense.

6.19 Why is the indirect fluorescent antibody (IFA) test performed?

The IFA test screens for HIV antibodies and is performed secondary to two positive ELISA tests.

6.20 Why is it difficult to detect HIV in a newborn?

Detecting HIV in a newborn is difficult because the newborn's blood still has HIV antibodies from either HIV-positive parent for 18 months.

6.21 What does the CD4+ count test measure?

The CD4+ count test measures the level of leukocytes to assess the patient's immune system.

6.22 What are the three types of leukocytes measured by the CD4+ test?

The three types of leukocytes (white blood cells, WBCs) important in fighting infection are T lymphocytes, T cells, and T-helper cells.

6.23 What is the purpose of the viral load measurement test?

The viral load measurement test is used to assess the progress and treatment of HIV infection by measuring the amount of HIV in the patient.

6.24 Why is the viral load measurement test administered when the patient is diagnosed with HIV?

A viral load measurement test is administered when the patient is diagnosed with HIV to establish the baseline.

6.25 What is the rheumatoid factor (RF)?

The RF is an autoantibody that destroys the patient's own tissues, resulting in stiffness, joint pain, and inflammation.

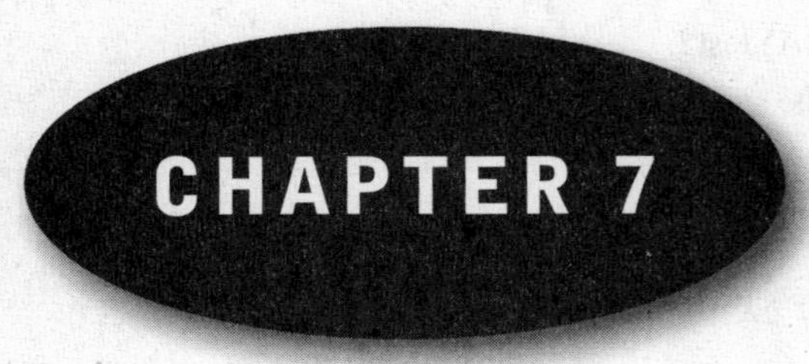

Endocrine Tests

7.1 Definition

The endocrine system transports hormones via blood vessels to regulate bodily functions, including metabolism, growth, mood, and tissue function. Hormones are created, stored, and released by glands and act as messengers, signaling other glands and organs to react in a specific manner.

Hormones are released based on existing hormone levels in the blood to maintain hormonal levels in balance. For example, an excess amount of a hormone may cause the release of a different hormone that causes the gland to stop or reduce excretion of the hormone, thereby bringing hormones in balance.

Diseases can alter the release of hormones, resulting in underproduction or overproduction of one or more hormones. Endocrine tests are administered to assess if the patient is experiencing an endocrine disease.

7.2 Adrenocorticotropic Hormone (ACTH) and Cortisol Test

The adrenocorticotropic hormone (ACTH) and cortisol test is used to assess the function of the pituitary gland and the adrenal glands.

Understanding the Adrenocorticotropic Hormone and Cortisol Test

The hypothalamus releases corticotropin-releasing hormone (CRH), which causes the pituitary gland to release the ACTH. Adrenocorticotropic hormone causes the adrenal gland to release cortisol. Cortisol increases blood pressure and glucose and reduces the immune responses. The ACTH test measures the level of ACTH in the blood. ACTH levels fall when cortisol levels rise, and ACTH level rise when cortisol levels fall.

The health care provider may request that an inferior petrosal sinus sample be taken from the inferior petrosal sinus near the pituitary gland to determine if the pituitary gland is producing ACTH or if ACTH is made elsewhere in the patient's body.

7.3 Overnight Dexamethasone Suppression Test

The overnight dexamethasone suppression test is used to assess the function of the adrenal glands and screen for Cushing's syndrome.

Understanding the Overnight Dexamethasone Suppression Test

The pituitary gland releases ACTH whenever there is a low level of cortisol in the blood. ACTH signals the adrenal glands to release cortisol. An adrenal gland tumor causes the release of cortisol in the absence of ACTH.

Dexamethasone is a medication similar to cortisol such that dexamethasone signals the pituitary gland that there is a high level of cortisol in the blood, causing the pituitary gland to suppress the release of ACTH.

The overnight dexamethasone suppression test examines the patient's cortisol level after dexamethasone is administered. The cortisol level should be lower because there is no ACTH in the blood to signal the adrenal glands to release cortisol. If cortisol levels remain high, then this is a sign of Cushing's syndrome as a result of an adrenal gland tumor producing cortisol.

7.4 Aldosterone Blood Test

The aldosterone blood test is used to screen for an adrenal gland tumor, an overactive adrenal gland, and the underlying cause of high blood pressure and low potassium levels in the blood.

Understanding the Aldosterone Blood Test

Kidneys release renin. Renin is a hormone that signals the adrenal glands to release aldosterone to control blood pressure and fluid and electrolytes balance by retaining fluid and sodium. The aldosterone test determines the level of aldosterone in the blood. This test is typically performed with the renin activity test.

7.5 Cortisol Blood Test

The cortisol blood test is used to assess the function of the pituitary and adrenal glands.

Understanding the Cortisol Blood Test

Cortisol, produced by the adrenal glands, is a hormone that causes an increase in blood pressure and an increase in glucose while decreasing the immune response. Cortisol levels reach their highest at 7 a.m. and their lowest 3 hours after sleep, which is based on the diurnal rhythm. However, the diurnal rhythm reverses if the patient works at night and sleeps during the day.

The pituitary gland releases ACTH whenever there is a low level of cortisol in the blood. ACTH signals the adrenal glands to release cortisol.

The health care provider may also order the dexamethasone suppression test, the adrenocorticotropic hormone test, or a 24-hour urine test.

7.6 Estrogen Blood Test

The estrogen blood test is used to assess the effect of fertility therapy and screen for abnormal sexual characteristics in men, estrogen-producing tumors, and fetal birth defects.

Understanding the Estrogen Blood Test

Estrogen is a hormone produced in the ovaries, placenta, muscle tissue, adipose tissue, adrenal glands, and testicles in men. There are three types of estrogen hormones:

1. **Estradiol:** Estrogen found in nonpregnant women that varies with the menstrual cycle.
2. **Estriol:** Estrogen that is produced by the placenta and is measured in pregnant women who are in at least the ninth week of pregnancy.
3. **Estrone:** Estrogen measured in women who have finished menopause, and in both men and women suggested of having testicular cancer, ovarian cancer, or adrenal gland tumor.

Estrogen levels can also be measured in urine. The health care provider may order a triple test or quad marker screen to assess for fetal birth defects. The maternal serum triple test measures levels of estrogen, alpha-fetoprotein (AFP), and human chorionic gonadotropin (hCG). The quad marker screen measures the same as the triple test, but also tests inhibit A hormone.

7.7 Growth Hormone (GH) Test

The growth hormone (GH) test is used to screen for abnormal growth and for pituitary gland tumors and to assess treatment.

Understanding the Growth Hormone Test

The human GH, secreted by the pituitary gland, stimulates cell growth and reproduction and growth factor 1 (IGF-1). The growth hormone test measures the level of growth hormone in blood.

The health care provider may order the growth factor 1 (IGF-1) test, the growth hormone suppression test (glucose loading test), and the growth hormone stimulation test (insulin tolerance test), along with the GH test.

7.8 Luteinizing Hormone (LH) Test

The luteinizing hormone (LH) test is used to assess the underlying cause of infertility or the effectiveness of infertility treatment, the underlying cause of irregular menstrual periods, or amenorrhea. In addition, this test also screens for menopause, the underlying cause of erectile dysfunction, and precocious and delayed puberty.

Understanding the Luteinizing Hormone Test

Luteinizing hormone is produced by the pituitary gland, which stimulates production of testosterone and ovulation, and regulates the menstrual cycle. Home ovulation testing kits detect LH levels in urine.

7.9 Parathyroid Hormone (PTH) Test

The parathyroid hormone (PTH) test is used to assess the underlying cause of abnormal calcium levels in the blood and screen for hyperparathyroidism.

Understanding the Parathyroid Hormone Test

The parathyroid glands release PTH when there is a low calcium level in the blood, causing the kidneys to retain calcium and bone to release calcium into the blood. Parathyroid hormone converts vitamin D to an active form, resulting in increased absorption of calcium by the intestine. Calcium and phosphorus have an inverse relationship. When the calcium level in blood is high, the phosphorus level in blood is low. Therefore, PTH also controls the phosphorus level in blood. The PTH test measures the level of PTH in blood.

The health care provider may also order tests for calcium and phosphorus levels in the blood and creatinine tests to assess kidney function.

7.10 Thyroid Hormone Test

The thyroid hormone tests are used to screen for hyper- and hypothyroidism and assess the treatment.

Understanding the Thyroid Hormone Tests

The hypothalamus gland releases thyrotropin-releasing hormone (TRH), which stimulates the anterior pituitary gland to release thyroid-stimulating hormone (TSH). Thyroid-stimulating hormone causes the thyroid gland to release thyroxine (T4) and triiodothyronine (T3), both of which regulate metabolism. T4 and T3 are produced only if there is sufficient iodine in the thyroid gland. T4 and T3 are transported in blood either freely or bound to globulin. Free T4 and T3 affect metabolism. The thyroid gland also releases calcitonin when the patient has hypercalcemia. Calcitonin regulates calcium levels in the blood by moving calcium from the blood to bone. The thyroid hormone tests measure the levels of T4 and T3 in the blood. There are four thyroid hormone tests:

1. **Total Thyroxine (T4):** This test measures the amount of T4 hormone that is bound to globulin and the amount of unbound T4 hormone, called free thyroxine, in the blood.
2. **Free Thyroxine (FT4):** This test measures the amount of unbound T4 hormone.
3. **Free Thyroxine Index (FTI):** This test compares the amount of bound thyroxine to total thyroxine, and thereby indirectly measures unbound thyroxine.
4. **Triiodothyronine (T3):** This test measures T3 hormone that is bound to globulin and the amount of unbound T3 hormone called free triiodothyronine.

7.11 Thyroid-Stimulating Hormone (TSH) Test

The thyroid-stimulating hormone (TSH) test is used to screen for hyper- and hypopituitarism and hypothalamus disorder. In addition, it is also used to screen for the underlying causes of hyper-and hypothyroidism and assess their treatment.

Understanding the Thyroid-Stimulating Hormone Test

The hypothalamus gland releases thyrotropin-releasing hormone (TRH), which stimulates the anterior pituitary gland to release TSH. Thyroid-stimulating hormone causes the thyroid gland to release thyroxine (T4) and triiodothyronine (T3), both of which regulate metabolism. The TSH test measures the level of TSH in the blood.

The health care provider will likely order thyroid hormone tests along with the TSH test.

7.12 Testosterone Test

The testosterone test is used to screen for the underlying causes of infertility, erectile dysfunction, osteoporosis in men, hirsutism in women, and irregular menstruation. It is also used to assess for precocious puberty in boys and assess treatment for prostate cancer.

Understanding the Testosterone Test

The pituitary gland releases luteinizing hormone that stimulates the release of testosterone by the adrenal glands, testes, and ovaries. Testosterone is unbound in blood, called *free* or ***bound*** to the sex hormone–binding globulin (SHBG) protein in blood. The testosterone test measures the level of testosterone in blood.

Solved Problems

Endocrine Tests

7.1 How do hormones work?

Hormones are created, stored, and released by glands and act as messengers signaling other glands and organs to react in a specific manner.

7.2 What is the purpose of the adrenocorticotropic hormone (ACTH) and cortisol tests?

The ACTH and cortisol tests are used to assess the function of the pituitary and adrenal glands.

7.3 What is the relationship between adrenocorticotropic hormone (ACTH) and cortisol?

ACTH levels fall when cortisol levels rise, and ACTH level rise when cortisol levels fall.

7.4 What is the impact of high cortisol levels in blood?

Cortisol increases blood pressure and glucose and reduces the immune responses.

7.5 What is the purpose of the overnight dexamethasone suppression test?

The overnight dexamethasone suppression test is used to assess the function of the adrenal glands and screen for Cushing's syndrome.

7.6 What is dexamethasone?

Dexamethasone is medication similar to cortisol in which dexamethasone signals to the pituitary gland that there is a high level of cortisol in the blood, causing the pituitary gland to suppress the release of ACTH.

7.7 What should happen when dexamethasone is administered?

The cortisol level should be lower because there is no ACTH in the blood to signal the adrenal glands to release cortisol. If cortisol levels remain high, this is a sign of Cushing's syndrome as a result of an adrenal gland tumor producing cortisol.

7.8 Why is the aldosterone blood test administered?

The aldosterone blood test is used to screen for an adrenal gland tumor, an overactive adrenal gland, and the underlying cause of high blood pressure and low potassium levels in the blood.

7.9 What is the relationship between aldosterone and renin?

Kidneys release renin. Renin is a hormone that signals the adrenal glands to release aldosterone to control blood pressure and fluid and electrolyte balance by retaining fluid and sodium.

7.10 Why is the estrogen blood test ordered?

The estrogen blood test is used to assess the affect of fertility therapy and screen for abnormal sexual characteristics in men, estrogen-producing tumors, and fetal birth defects

7.11 What is estradiol?

Estradiol is estrogen found in nonpregnant women that varies with the menstrual cycle.

7.12 What is estriol?

Estriol is estrogen that is produced by the placenta and is measured in pregnant women who are in at least the ninth week of pregnancy.

7.13 What is estrone?

Estrone is estrogen measured in women who have finished menopause, and in both men and women suggested of having testicular cancer, ovarian cancer, or an adrenal gland tumor.

7.14 Why might a health care provider measure growth hormone (GH)?

The GH test is used to assess treatment for abnormal growth and screen for abnormal growth and a pituitary gland tumor.

7.15 Where is GH secreted?

The human GH, secreted by the pituitary gland, stimulates cell growth and reproduction and growth factor 1 (IGF-1).

7.16 What is the purpose of the luteinizing hormone (LH) test?

The LH test is used to assess the underlying cause of infertility or the effectiveness of infertility treatment, the underlying cause of irregular menstrual periods, or amenorrhea. It is also used to screen for menopause, the underlying cause of erectile dysfunction, and precocious and delayed puberty.

7.17 What is the function of (LH)?

Luteinizing hormone is produced by the pituitary gland, which stimulates the production of testosterone and ovulation and regulates the menstrual cycle.

7.18 Why would a health care provider order the parathyroid hormone (PTH) test?

The PTH test is used to assess the underlying cause of an abnormal calcium level in the blood and screen for hyperparathyroidism.

7.19 What is the relationship between the PTH and calcium level in the blood?

The parathyroid glands release PTH when the calcium level in the blood is low, causing the kidneys to retain calcium and bone to release calcium into the blood. Parathyroid hormone converts vitamin D to an active form, resulting in increased absorption of calcium by the intestine.

7.20 How does the PTH control the phosphorus level in the blood?

Calcium and phosphorus have an inverse relationship. When the calcium level in the blood is high, the phosphorus level in the blood is low. Therefore, PTH also controls the phosphorus level in the blood.

7.21 Why is the thyroid hormone test administered?

The thyroid hormone test is used to screen for hyper- and hypothyroidism and assess for their treatment.

7.22 What is the relationship between the hypothalamus gland and the thyroid gland?

The hypothalamus gland releases thyrotropin-releasing hormone (TRH), which stimulates the anterior pituitary gland to release thyroid-stimulating hormone (TSH). Thyroid-stimulating hormone causes the thyroid gland to release thyroxine (T4) and triiodothyronine (T3), both of which regulate metabolism.

7.23 What is the function of calcitonin?

The thyroid gland also releases calcitonin when the patient has hypercalcemia. Calcitonin regulates calcium levels in the blood by moving calcium from the blood to the bone.

7.24 Why might the health care provider order the thyroid-stimulating hormone (TSH) test?

The TSH test is used to screen for hyper- and hypopituitarism and hypothalamus disorder. It is also used to screen for the underlying causes of hyper- and hypothyroidism and assess their treatment.

7.25 What is the relationship between luteinizing hormone (LH) and testosterone?

The pituitary gland releases LH, which stimulates the release of testosterone by the adrenal glands, testes, and ovaries.

Glucose Tests

8.1 Definition

There are two pancreatic endocrine hormones secreted by the islet cells in the pancreas. These are *insulin* and *glucagon*. Both are secreted based on blood glucose levels. When the blood glucose is elevated, the pancreas secretes insulin, which causes glucose to cross the cell membrane and allows it to be used for energy, resulting in a decrease in blood glucose.

When blood glucose levels are low, the pancreas secretes glucagon, which signals the liver to release stored glucose into the blood, resulting in an increase in blood glucose. Other cells such as muscles also release glucose in response to glucagon.

Blood glucose must be maintained within a narrow range, which occurs naturally with the secretion of insulin and glucagon. However, failure of islet cells to properly function due to diseases such as diabetes, can result in high levels of blood glucose (hyperglycemia) or low levels of blood glucose (hypoglycemia).

Health care providers order glucose tests to monitor the blood glucose level. Based on the results of these tests, the health care provider may administer insulin or glucose to the patient.

8.2 C-Peptide Test

The C-peptide test to is used to differentiate between type 1 and type 2 diabetes and is used to assess the underlying cause of hypoglycemia and the result of removing an insulinoma (tumor) from the pancreas.

Understanding the C-Peptide Test

Proinsulin is the precursor to insulin produced by the beta cells of the islets of Langerhans in the pancreas. Proinsulin is split into C-peptide and insulin. The level of C-peptide is considered equal to the amount of insulin, indicating the amount of insulin made by the pancreas. The C-peptide test measures the level of C-peptide in blood and is used to differentiate between type 1 and type 2 diabetes.

The health care provider will order a blood glucose test along with the C-peptide test. The health care provider may order a C-peptide stimulation test to differentiate between type 1 and type 2 diabetes.

8.3 D-Xylose Absorption Test

The D-xylose absorption test is used to screen for malabsorption syndrome.

Understanding the D-Xylose Absorption Test

D-xylose is a simple sugar that is absorbed by the intestine. The D-xylose absorption test measures the level of D-xylose in blood.

D-xylose absorption can also be tested with a urine sample; however, a urine test is less accurate than the blood D-xylose absorption test for patients <12 years of age. The health care provider may order an upper gastrointestinal series if the D-xylose test is positive.

8.4 Blood Glucose Test

Blood glucose tests are used to screen for diabetes and hypoglycemia and assess treatment for diabetes.

Understanding Blood Glucose Tests

Glucose is the source of energy for cells and is transported into cells by insulin. As blood glucose levels rise following ingestion of food, the pancreas releases insulin to move the glucose from blood into cells. Blood glucose tests measure the level of glucose in the blood. There are four blood glucose tests:

1. **Oral Glucose Tolerance Test (OGTT):** This test measures the blood glucose levels at specific time intervals after the patient ingests a glucose drink. The OGTT is ordered to screen for gestational diabetes and confirm positive results of other blood glucose tests.
2. **2-Hour Postprandial Blood Sugar:** This test measures blood glucose levels 2 hours after the patient ingests food.
3. **Fasting Blood Sugar (FBS):** This test measures blood glucose levels after the patient has fasted for 8 hours. The FBS test is the initial test for diabetes.
4. **Random Blood Sugar (RBS):** This test measures blood glucose levels several times a day regardless of food intake.

Glucose levels can also be measured in urine; however, this is not used to diagnose or monitor glucose levels. The health care provider may order the glycohemoglobin (GHb) blood test, which is used to monitor blood glucose levels for the previous 120 days.

8.5 Glycohemoglobin (GHb) Test

The glycohemoglobin (GHb) test is used to assess the treatment for diabetes and assess if the patient is adhering to the treatment plan.

Understanding the Glycohemoglobin Test

Glucose binds to hemoglobin in red blood cells, which has a life span of 120 days. The glycohemoglobin (GHb) test, commonly known as HgbA1c, measures the level of glucose bound to hemoglobin. This differs from the blood glucose test that measures the level of glucose in plasma. The health care provider orders the GHb test to assess if treatment is controlling diabetes and the patient is adhering to the treatment over a 120-day period.

The GHb test can be administered at any time; however, the health care provider is likely to order the test four times a year. The GHb test is not a replacement for the blood glucose test and cannot dictate hypoglycemia.

Solved Problems

Glucose Tests

8.1 Where is glucagon produced?

Glucagon is produced by the islet cells in the pancreas.

8.2 How do insulin and glucagon affect the blood glucose level?

When blood glucose is elevated, the pancreas secretes insulin, which causes glucose to cross the cell membrane and allows it to be used for energy, resulting in a decrease in blood glucose.

When blood glucose levels are low, the pancreas secretes glucagon, which signals the liver to release stored glucose into the blood, resulting in an increase in blood glucose.

8.3 What happens if the islet cells fail to properly function?

Failure of islet cells to properly function because of diseases such as diabetes can result in high levels of blood glucose (hyperglycemia) or low levels of blood glucose (hypoglycemia).

8.4 What is a cause of hypoglycemia?

Too much insulin is a cause of hypoglycemia.

8.5 What is the function of an insulinoma?

An insulinoma is a tumor that produces insulin.

8.6 What is the purpose of the C-peptide test?

The C-peptide test to is used to differentiate between type 1 and type 2 diabetes, and is used to assess the underlying cause of hypoglycemia, as well as the result of removing an insulinoma (tumor) from the pancreas.

8.7 How does the C-peptide test differentiate between type 1 and type 2 diabetes?

Proinsulin is the precursor to insulin produced by the beta cells of the islets of Langerhans in the pancreas. Proinsulin is split into C-peptide and insulin. The level of C-peptide is considered equal to the amount of insulin, indicating the amount of insulin made by the pancreas.

8.8 What is D-xylose?

D-xylose is a simple sugar that is absorbed by the intestine.

8.9 What is the purpose of the D-xylose absorption test?

The D-xylose absorption test is used to screen for malabsorption syndrome.

8.10 What might you expect the health care provider to order if the D-xylose absorption test is positive?

The health care provider may order an upper gastrointestinal series if the D-xylose test is positive.

8.11 Why would a health care provider not order a D-xylose urine test for a patient who is 10 years old?

D-xylose absorption can also be tested with a urine sample. Urine test is less accurate than the blood D-xylose absorption test for patients <12 years of age.

8.12 What might the health care provider order along with the C-peptide test?

The health care provider might order a blood glucose test along with the C-peptide test.

8.13 What is the purpose of a blood glucose test?

The blood glucose test is used to screen for diabetes and hypoglycemia and assess treatment for diabetes.

8.14 What is a common reason there is an increase in insulin production?

Ingestion of food is a common reason for an increase in insulin production.

8.15 What is the oral glucose tolerance (OGTT) test?

The OGTT measures the blood glucose levels at specific time intervals after the patient ingests a glucose drink. The OGTT test is ordered to screen for gestational diabetes and confirm positive results of other blood glucose tests.

8.16 What is the 2-hour postprandial blood sugar test?

The 2-hour postprandial blood sugar test measures blood glucose levels 2 hours after the patient ingests food.

8.17 What is the fasting blood sugar (FBS) test?

The FBS test measures blood glucose levels after the patient has fasted for 8 hours. The FBS test is the initial test for diabetes.

8.18 What is the random blood sugar (RBS) test?

The RBS test measures blood glucose levels several times a day regardless of food intake.

8.19 Why would the health care provider not order glucose levels to be measured in urine?

Glucose levels can be measured in urine; however, this is not used to diagnose or monitor glucose levels.

8.20 What is the purpose of the glycohemoglobin (GHb) test?

The GHb test is used to assess the treatment for diabetes and assess if the patient is adhering to the treatment plan.

8.21 Where in the blood does glucose bind?

Glucose binds to hemoglobin in red blood cells (RBCs).

8.22 Why does the result of the GHb test represent the patient's condition for the previous 120 days?

Red blood cells have a life span of 120 days.

8.23 How does the GHb test differ from the blood glucose test?

The GHb test measures glucose bound to hemoglobin in RBCs. The blood glucose test measures glucose in plasma.

8.24 When is the health care provider likely to order the GHb test?

The GHb test can be administered at any time; however, the health care provider is likely to order the test four times a year.

8.25 For what is the GHb test unable to screen?

The GHb test is unable to screen for hypoglycemia.

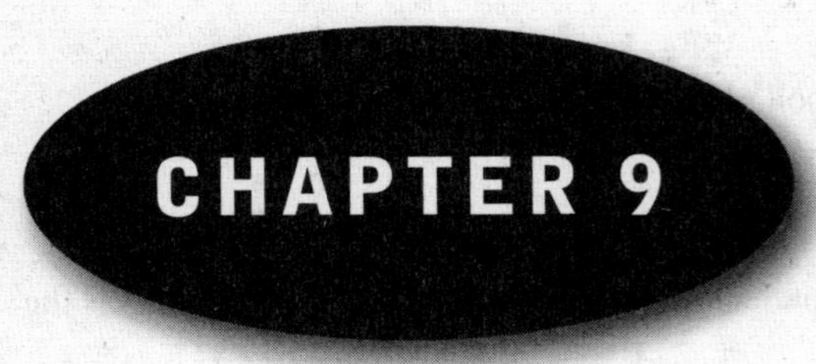

Tumor Markers

9.1 Definition

A tumor is an uncontrollable growth of cells that may be malignant (cancerous) or benign (noncancerous). Blood tests are performed to detect the presence of tumor markers. A tumor marker is a substance, usually a protein, produced either by tumor cells or other cells in response to the presence of the tumor.

The presence of a tumor marker does not mean that the patient has cancer. Conditions other than cancer can also generate a tumor marker. Likewise, the absence of a tumor marker does not mean that the patient is cancer free, because many times early stages of cancer do not produce a tumor marker.

In addition to tumor markers, a patient's blood can also be tested for cancer genomics. Cancer genomics are mutations of specific genes, which are called risk markers. A risk marker indicates that a patient has a higher than normal risk for developing cancer, although there is not yet a sign of cancer. Conversely, the presence of the tumor marker indicates the possibility that a tumor is present.

9.2 Cancer Antigen 125 (CA-125) Test

The cancer antigen 125 (CA-125) test is used to screen for ovarian cancer and other types of cancer. It is also used to assess the effectiveness of cancer treatment.

Understanding the Cancer Antigen 125 Test

Cancer antigen 125 is a protein attached to ovarian cancer cells and other cancer cells. The CA-125 test measures the level of CA-125 in the blood.

The CA-125 test is not used to differentiate between a benign or malignant ovarian tumor. The health care provider may order testing of peritoneal fluid and the chest to assess if CA-125 is present.

9.3 Carcinoembryonic Antigen (CEA) Test

The carcinoembryonic antigen (CEA) test is used screen for cancer. It is also used to assess the effectiveness of cancer treatment and the success of surgical removal of the cancer.

Understanding the Carcinoembryonic Antigen Test

The carcinoembryonic antigen is a protein present during fetal development that terminates at birth. The CEA is produced in certain types of cancers. The CEA test measures the level of carcinoembryonic antigen in blood.

CEA is not used to screen for early detection of a cancer and is not used to diagnose cancer. Most cancers do not cause high levels of CEA. The health care provider may order tests of peritoneal fluid and cerebrospinal fluid to determine if the cancer metastasized.

9.4 Prostate-Specific Antigen (PSA) Test

The prostate-specific antigen (PSA) test is used screen for prostate cancer. It is also used to assess the effectiveness of prostate cancer treatment.

Understanding the Prostate-Specific Antigen Test

The prostate gland releases prostate-specific antigen in low amounts. Increased amounts are released with an enlarged prostate gland, prostatitis, prostate cancer, and from injury resulting from a digital rectal exam, cystoscopy, or sexual activity. The PSA test measures the level of prostate-specific antigen in blood. The PSA level can be normal in a patient who has prostate cancer.

The PSA test is performed in conjunction with a digital rectal examination.

- **Prostate-Specific Antigen Density (PSAD) Test:** This test compares the PSA value with the prostate gland size.
- **Prostate-Specific Antigen Velocity Test:** This test determines if the PSA has increased over time.
- **Complex Prostate-Specific Antigen (cPSA) Test:** This test detects prostate cancer.
- **Transrectal Ultrasound (TRUS) Test:** This test measures the size of the prostate gland.

Solved Problems

Tumor Markers

9.1 What is a tumor?

A tumor is an uncontrollable growth of cells.

9.2 What is a malignant tumor?

A malignant tumor is a cancerous tumor.

9.3 What is a benign tumor?

A benign tumor is a noncancerous tumor.

9.4 What is a tumor marker?

A tumor marker is a substance, usually a protein, that is produced either by tumor cells or other cells in response to the presence of a tumor.

9.5 Does the presence of a tumor marker mean that the patient has cancer?

No. Other conditions can also generate a tumor marker.

9.6 Does the absence of a tumor marker mean that the patient is free from cancer?

No. Many times early stages of cancer do not produce a tumor marker.

9.7 What are cancer genomics?

Cancer genomics are mutations of specific genes.

9.8 What is a risk marker?

A risk marker indicates that a patient has a higher than normal risk for developing cancer.

9.9 Does the patient have cancer if a positive risk marker is present?

No. The risk marker indicates there is a cancer genomics present that increases the risk for cancer but there is no sign of cancer.

9.10 What is cancer antigen 125 (CA-125)?

CA-125 is a protein attached to the ovarian cancer cells and other cancer cells.

9.11 What is the purpose of the CA-125 test?

The CA-125 test is used screen for ovarian cancer and other types of cancer. It is also used to assess the effectiveness of cancer treatment.

9.12 Does the CA-125 test determine if an ovarian tumor is malignant?

The CA-125 test is not used to differentiate between a benign or malignant ovarian tumor.

9.13 If the CA-125 test is positive, what other testing may a health care provider order?

The health care provider may order testing of peritoneal fluid and the chest to assess if cancer antigen 125 is present.

9.14 What is the carcinoembryonic antigen (CEA)?

The CEA is a protein present during fetal development that terminates at birth.

9.15 What is the purpose of the CEA test?

The CEA test is used to screen for cancer. It is also used to assess the effectiveness of cancer treatment and the success of surgical removal of the cancer.

9.16 Why is the CEA test not used for diagnosis of cancer?

Most cancers do not cause high levels of the carcinoembryonic antigen.

9.17 What might the health care provider order to determine if cancer metastasized?

The health care provider may order test of peritoneal fluid and cerebrospinal fluid to determine if the cancer metastasized.

9.18 What is the purpose of the prostate-specific antigen (PSA) test?

The PSA test is used screen for prostate cancer. It is also used to assess the effectiveness of prostate cancer treatment.

9.19 How would you respond if the patient said that his friend's PSA level was low?

The prostate gland releases PSA in low amounts.

9.20 How would you respond if the patient said that he has prostate cancer because the PSA level is high?

Increased amounts are released with an enlarged prostate gland, prostatitis, and prostate cancer, and from injury resulting from a digital rectal exam, cystoscopy, or sexual activity.

9.21 How would you respond if a patient says he does not have prostate cancer because his PSA level is normal?

The PSA level can be normal in a patient who has prostate cancer.

9.22 **Why would a health care provider order a prostate-specific antigen density (PSAD) test?**
The health care provider may also order the PSAD test to compare the PSA value to the prostate gland size.

9.23 **Why would be health care provider order a prostate-specific antigen velocity test?**
The health care provider would order a prostate-specific antigen velocity test to determine if PSA increases over time.

9.24 **Why would the health care provider order the complex prostate-specific antigen (cPSA) test?**
The health care provider would order the cPSA test to detect prostate cancer.

9.25 **Why would the health care provider order the transrectal ultrasound (TRUS) test?**
The TRUS test measures the size of the prostate gland.

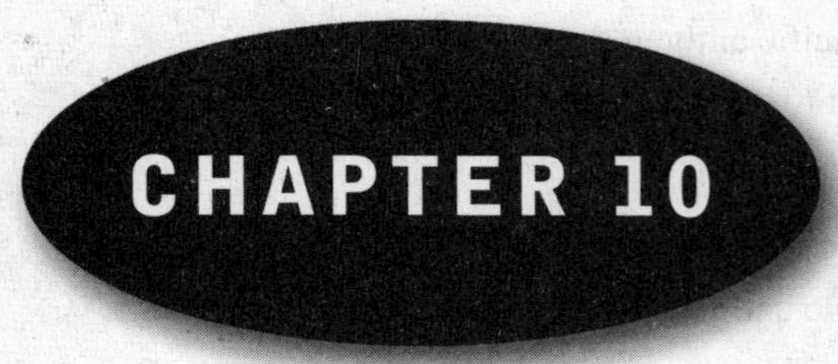

Pregnancy and Genetics Tests

10.1 Definition

Health care providers have an arsenal of tests that provide clues to the underlying cause of infertility and risk for genetic disorders that can affect the fetus or newborn. There are screening tests whose purpose is to assess if the patient is at risk for a disease, and diagnostic tests that are used to determine if the patient has a disease. These tests are ordered to screen patients for disorders when there are no telltale signs or symptoms and other tests are ordered when the health care provider is looking to confirm a sign or symptom that something is outside the normal parameters.

These tests look for certain components in blood such as the presence of antibodies or certain enzymes or the levels of protein and hormones. Scientific research has determined that the absence or existence of these components in blood correlates to the presence or absence of a specific disorder.

10.2 Antisperm Antibody Test

The antisperm antibody test is used to assess if antisperm antibodies are in blood, vaginal fluid, or semen, and assess the underlying cause of infertility.

Understanding the Antisperm Antibody Test

An immune system response can be caused by semen resulting in antibodies attaching to and killing sperm, causing immunologic infertility. These antibodies can be in blood, vaginal fluids, or semen. Antibodies can be made in a male if his sperm comes in contact with his immune system as a result of testicular injury, prostate gland infection, vasectomy, or other surgeries that expose sperm to the immune system. Semen in sperm can cause an allergic reaction in a female partner.

Some health care providers question the usefulness of the test since treatment is the same regardless of the test results.

10.3 Alpha-Fetoprotein (AFP) Test

The alpha-fetoprotein (AFP) test is used to assess:

- Fetal neural tube defects
- Spina bifida
- Anencephaly

- Edward's syndrome (trisomy 18)
- Down's syndrome (trisomy 21)
- Omphalocele
- Hepatoma in patients who have chronic hepatitis B or cirrhosis
- Lymphoma
- Hodgkin's disease
- Renal cell cancer
- Ovarian cancer
- Testicular cancer
- Pancreatic cancer
- Effectiveness of cancer treatment

Understanding the Alpha-Fetoprotein Test

Alpha-fetoprotein is produced by the fetal liver and is detectable in a pregnant woman's blood. The level of AFP rises gradually in the fourteenth week of gestation and continues rising until around the thirty-fourth week of gestation when the AFP level gradually decreases.

A high or low level of AFP is a sign that there may be a problem with fetal development. The AFP test is commonly administered as part of a maternal serum triple or quadruple screening test, which along with other factors including the pregnant woman's age, is used to estimate the chance of birth defects.

The maternal serum triple screening test examines levels of:

- Alpha-fetoprotein
- Beta human chorionic gonadotropin (beta-hCG)
- Unconjugated estriol or uE3 (estrogen)

The maternal serum quadruple screening test examines levels of:

- The same substance as the maternal serum triple screening test
- The hormone inhibin A

A health care provider may also administer the AFP test in nonpregnant women and children and men to assess for a number of other diseases that cause a high level of AFP in the blood. These include lymphoma, Hodgkin's disease, ovarian cancer, testicular cancer, renal cell cancer, and pancreatic cancer. Half of patients diagnosed with these cancers have normal AFP test results.

10.4 Follicle-Stimulating Hormone (FSH) Test

The follicle-stimulating hormone (FSH) test is used to assess the underlying cause of infertility and abnormal menstrual periods. It is also used to assess for precocious puberty, abnormal development of sexual organs, and the function of the pituitary gland.

Understanding the Follicle-Stimulating Hormone Test

The follicle-stimulating hormone is produced by the pituitary gland and controls sperm production by the testes and egg production in the ovaries. Follicle-stimulating hormone level is constant in men and changes with the menstrual cycle in women, with the highest level occurring during ovulation. The FSH test measures the level of the FSH in blood.

The health care provider may order the luteinizing hormone (LH) blood test, estrogen blood test, and the progesterone blood test in addition to the FSH test. The health care provider may order a sperm count or assessment of the patient's ovarian reserve.

10.5 Human Chorionic Gonadotropin (hCG) Test

The human chorionic gonadotropin (hCG) test is used to assess for:

- Pregnancy
- Ectopic pregnancy
- Molar pregnancy
- Treatment for molar pregnancy
- Testicular cancer
- Choriocarcinoma

Understanding the Human Chorionic Gonadotropin Test

When a fertilized egg implants to the uterine wall, the placenta begins development. By the ninth day, the placenta produces the hCG hormone, which is detectable in the patient's blood. The hCG test measures the level of hCG in blood. The level of hCG hormone is used as a sign of pregnancy, which is confirmed by other tests. In a normal pregnancy, the level of hCG hormone increases until 16 weeks' gestation and then gradually decreases until birth when no hCG hormone is detectable. A lower level of hCG hormone might indicate an ectopic pregnancy and a higher level may indicate multiple fetuses. The hCG hormone test is typically ordered as part of a maternal serum screening test that is administered at 15 weeks' gestation.

The hCG hormone can also be produced by a molar pregnancy, choriocarcinoma (uterine cancer), ovarian cancer, or other tumors. Testicular cancer also produces the hCG hormone in men. A normal hCG hormone level does not rule out cancer.

The level of hCG hormone can be detected before the patient misses her menstrual period and as early as 6 days after attachment of the egg. The hCG hormone test is also available as a urine test (home pregnancy test), which determines if the hCG hormone is present but does not measure the hormone's level. The hCG hormone level is high 4 weeks following an abortion.

10.6 Inhibin A Test

The inhibin A test is used to assess the risk of Down's syndrome and other birth defects.

Understanding the Inhibin A Test

Inhibin A hormone is secreted by the placenta and the level of the hormone is measured by the hormone inhibin A test. The hormone inhibin A test is a component of the quadruple screen test that is administered at the twentieth week of gestation to determine if there is a risk of birth defect in the fetus such as Down's syndrome. The quad screen test also includes the AFP test, beta human chorionic gonadotropin (beta-hCG) test, and the uE3 test.

The hormone inhibin A test is not used to diagnose potential birth defects. Further testing is required if the hormone inhibin A test is abnormal.

10.7 Prolactin Test

The prolactin test is used to assess:

- Prolactinoma (pituitary gland tumor)
- Underlying cause of amenorrhea
- Underlying cause of infertility
- Underlying cause of nipple discharge
- Erectile dysfunction

Understanding the Prolactin Test

Prolactin is a hormone produced by the pituitary gland that increases during pregnancy, causing an increase in milk production and enlargement of the mammary glands. A high level of progesterone that occurs during pregnancy prevents milk from ejecting. Progesterone levels fall after delivery. As the newborn sucks the nipple to cause ejection of milk from the breast, this action simulates release of prolactin, causing lactogenesis and resulting in increased production of milk. Prolactin levels return to normal after delivery if the mother is not breast-feeding. The prolactin test measures the level of prolactin in the blood.

10.8 Phenylketonuria (PKU) Test

The phenylketonuria (PKU) test is used to assess for phenylketonuria.

Understanding the Phenylketonuria Test

Phenylalanine is an amino acid in breast milk, formula, dairy products, and meats. The body requires the phenylalanine hydroxylase enzyme to metabolize phenylalanine into tyrosine. Phenylketonuria is a genetic disorder in which the patient is missing the phenylalanine hydroxylase enzyme and is therefore unable to metabolize phenylalanine, causing a buildup of phenylalanine level in the blood that results in mental retardation and seizures. The PKU test measures the level of the phenylalanine hydroxylase enzyme in blood. The PKU test is administered to newborns between 12 and 28 hours after birth and again a week after birth.

Infants older than 6 weeks of age may be administered a PKU test if it was not performed at birth. Newborns who are ill are retested 3 weeks after birth.

10.9 Tay-Sachs Test

The Tay-Sachs test is used to assess for Tay-Sachs disease and if the patient is carrying the Tay-Sachs trait.

Understanding the Tay-Sachs Test

Hexosaminidase A is an enzyme that metabolizes ganglioside, which is a fatty acid. If hexosaminidase A is not present, ganglioside accumulates in brain and nerve cells, resulting in neural damage. This is referred to as Tay-Sachs disease, which is an inherited disease. The Tay-Sachs test measures the amount of hexosaminidase A in the blood.

A positive result will be confirmed by genetic testing.

The health care provider may order an amniocentesis or chorionic villus sampling of the placenta to determine if the fetus has the hexosaminidase A enzyme.

10.10 Sickle Cell Test

The sickle cell test is used to assess for sickle cell disease and if the patient is carrying the sickle cell trait.

Understanding the Sickle Cell Test

Normal red blood cells (RBCs) contain hemoglobin A. In sickle cell disease, RBCs contain hemoglobin S, which causes the RBC to form a sickle shape and is therefore called a sickled blood cell. Sickle cell disease is an autosomal recessive disease in which the sickle cell gene must be inherited from both parents. Patients with sickled blood cells can experience a sickle cell crisis when sickled blood cells block blood vessels, resulting in decreased blood flow. Sickled blood cells are destroyed faster than normal RBCs, leading to sickle cell anemia. The sickle cell test determines if the patient has sickled blood cells.

The patient should undergo genetic counseling if the patient has the sickle cell trait or sickle cell disease.

The health care provider may order the high-performance liquid chromatography (HPLC) test to examine the patient's DNA for the sickle cell gene. Sickle cell disease is more prevalent in African Americans. Health care providers commonly test newborns for the sickle cell trait, although infants <6 months old can have false-negative test results since they have fetal hemoglobin in their blood. The sickle cell test is therefore repeated after 6 months of age. The health care provider may order the sickle cell test for a fetus using chorionic villus sampling (CVS) or amniocentesis.

10.11 Hemochromatosis (HFE) Gene Test

The hemochromatosis (HFE) gene test is used to screen for the HFE gene and assesses the underlying cause and treatment of HFE.

Understanding the Hemochromatosis Gene Test

The hemochromatosis gene increases the absorption of iron (hemochromatosis), which causes a buildup of iron in the liver, heart, blood, joints, skin, and pancreas and results in joint pain, weight loss, and decreased energy. This can lead to arrhythmia, cirrhosis, diabetes, heart failure, arthritis, and change in skin color. The HFE gene test determines if the patient has the HFE gene.

Existence of the HFE gene means that the patient has an increased chance of having HFE, but does not mean that the patient has HFE. It is advised that the patient consult a genetic counselor before the test is administered to discuss the risks of developing HFE.

The health care provider will order the test if close family members have HFE. The health care provider might order the ferritin level test and transferring saturation test to measure the level of iron in the patient's blood.

Solved Problems

Pregnancy and Genetic Tests

10.1 What is the purpose of the antisperm antibody test?

The antisperm antibody test is used to assess if antisperm antibodies are in blood, vaginal fluid, or semen, and to assess the underlying cause of infertility.

10.2 How might the immune system kill sperm?

An immune system response can be caused by semen resulting in antibodies attaching to and killing sperm, causing immunologic infertility.

10.3 Where are antisperm antibodies located?

These antibodies can be in blood, vaginal fluids, or semen.

10.4 How can antisperm antibodies be made?

Antibodies can be made in a male if his sperm comes in contact with his immune system as a result of testicular injury, prostate gland infection, vasectomy, or other surgeries that expose sperm to the immune system.

10.5 Why might the health care provider not order the antisperm antibodies test?

Some health care providers question the usefulness of the test since treatment is the same regardless of the test results.

10.6 What is the purpose of the alpha-fetoprotein (AFP) test?

The AFP test is used to assess for fetal neural tube defects, spinal bifida, anencephaly, Edward's syndrome (trisomy 18), Down's syndrome (trisomy 21), omphalocele, hepatoma in patients who have chronic hepatitis B or cirrhosis, lymphoma, Hodgkin's disease, renal cell cancer, ovarian cancer, testicular cancer, pancreatic cancer, and effectiveness of cancer treatment.

10.7 Where is AFP produced?

AFP is produced by the fetal liver and is detectable in a pregnant woman's blood.

10.8 What might a high or low AFP level indicate?

A high or low level of AFP is a sign that there may be a problem with fetal development.

10.9 Of what does the maternal serum triple screen test consist?

The maternal serum triple screening test examines levels of AFP, beta human chorionic gonadotropin (beta-hCG), and unconjugated estriol or uE3 (estrogen).

10.10 Why might a health care provider order the follicle-stimulating hormone (FSH) test?

The FSH test is used to assess the underlying cause of infertility and abnormal menstrual periods. It is also used to assess for precocious puberty, abnormal development of sexual organs, and to assess the function of the pituitary gland.

10.11 What is the function of FSH?

The FSH is produced by the pituitary gland and controls sperm production by the testes and egg production in the ovaries.

10.12 Is the FSH level normally constant?

The FSH level is constant in men and changes with the menstrual cycle in women, with the highest level occurring during ovulation.

10.13 What other test might a health care provider order along with the FSH test?

The health care provider may order the luteinizing hormone (LH) blood test, estrogen blood test, and the progesterone blood test in addition to the FSH test.

10.14 Why might the health care provider order the human chorionic gonadotropin (hCG) test?

The human chorionic gonadotropin (hCG) test is used to assess for pregnancy, ectopic and molar pregnancy, treatment for molar pregnancy, testicular cancer, and choriocarcinoma.

10.15 Why is the hCG test administered to determine pregnancy?

When a fertilized egg implants to the uterine wall, the placenta begins to develop. By the ninth day, the placenta produces hCG hormone, which is detectable in the patient's blood.

10.16 Is the hCG test used to determine if the patient is pregnant?

No. Additional tests are necessary to confirm a pregnancy.

10.17 What might a low level of hGC indicate?

A low level of hCG hormone might indicate an ectopic pregnancy, and a high level might indicate multiple fetuses.

10.18 When is the peak period for hCG?

In a normal pregnancy, the level of the hCG hormone increases until 16 weeks' gestation and then gradually decreases until birth when no hCG hormone is detectable.

10.19 What else besides pregnancy can produce hCG?

The hCG hormone can also be produced by a molar pregnancy, choriocarcinoma (uterine cancer), ovarian cancer, or other tumors.

10.20 Can hCG be produced in men?

Testicular cancer also produces the hCG hormone in men.

10.21 What is the purpose of the inhibin A test?

The inhibin A test is used to assess the risk of Down's syndrome and other birth defects.

10.22 When is the inhibin A test administered?

The inhibin A hormone test is a component of the quad screen tests that is administered at the twentieth week of gestation.

10.23 Is the inhibit A test used to diagnose potential birth defects?

No. Further testing is necessary before a diagnosis is reached.

10.24 Why is the prolactin test ordered?

The prolactin test is used to assess for prolactinoma (pituitary gland tumor), the underlying cause of amenorrhea, infertility, and nipple discharge, and erectile dysfunction.

10.25 What is prolactin?

Prolactin is a hormone produced by the pituitary gland that increases during pregnancy, causing an increase in milk production and enlargement of the mammary glands.

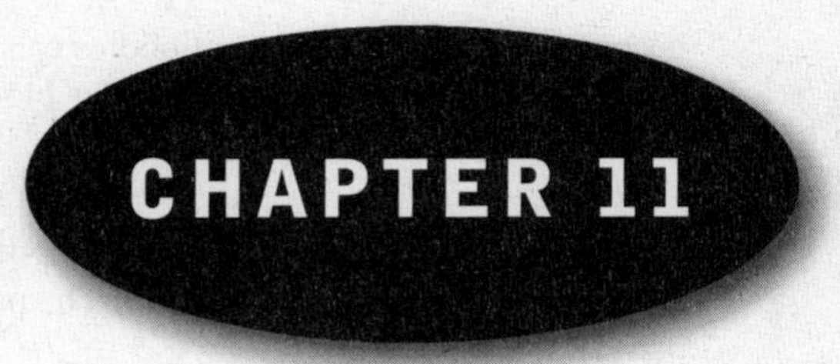

Tests for Infection

11.1 Definition

Signs and symptoms of an infection typically indicate that a microorganism has invaded the patient's body. There has been a tendency for health care providers to prescribe an antibiotic at the first sign of an infection. In doing so, the health care provider assumes that the patient is experiencing a bacterial infection and that the antibiotic will eliminate the bacteria. Typically, if the infection does not improve within 7 to 10 days of antibiotic treatment, the patient will undergo an additional assessment.

Over time, this approach to treating infection has been one of many factors leading to antibiotic-resistant bacteria. The bacteria adapted to common antibiotics, making the antibiotic useless. Today health care providers are encouraged to order tests that identify the microorganism as well as tests to identify the best medication to kill the microorganism. These tests are called culture and sensitivity tests.

A sample of the patient's blood or infected tissue is sent to the laboratory, where the microorganism is encouraged to replicate in a culture dish. Laboratory specialists then conduct tests to identify the microorganism. Once identified, the microorganism is exposed to medication known to kill it. The laboratory specialist determines the best medication and the minimum dose to administer to the patient that will kill the microorganism. In this way, the proper dose of the right medication can be prescribed, reducing the risk that the microorganism will become resistant to the medication.

11.2 Antibody Tests

Antibody tests are used to assess the underlying cause of autoimmune hemolytic anemia, blood transfusion reaction, or potential reaction, and screen for the Rh factor.

Understanding Antibody Tests

Antibodies are proteins made by the immune system that bind to bacteria, viruses, and other microorganisms to destroy the microorganism. Antibodies can also bind to red blood cells (RBCs), destroying them as well. Antibody tests determine if antibodies are attacking RBCs. Antibodies are created as a result of:

- **Blood Transfusion Reaction:** The transfused blood has different antigens on the surface of its RBCs than the patient's RBCs, which causes the immune system to produce antibodies that attack the transfused RBCs.
- **Rhesus Factor Sensitization:** The Rh antigen is in the fetus's blood (Rh positive), but not in the pregnant woman's blood (Rh negative). During delivery, the fetus's blood mixes with the mother's blood, causing the mother's immune system to create antibodies against the fetus's RBCs. The mother

becomes Rh sensitive. The antibodies can attack the fetus's RBCs in future pregnancies if the fetus is Rh positive. Women with Rh-negative blood are given the Rh immune globulin (RhoGAM) that typically stops Rh sensitivity.

  - *Rh Antibody Titer:* The test is performed in early pregnancy to determine the mother's blood type and conclude if the mother is Rh negative.

- **Autoimmune Hemolytic Anemia:** The patient's immune system creates antibodies against the patient's RBCs.
  - *Direct Coombs Test:* Identifies antibodies attached to the patient's RBCs. This test is performed:
    - On a newborn whose mother is Rh negative to determine if the antibodies crossed the placenta into the newborn's blood
    - On a patient who received a blood transfusion to determine if there is a transfusion reaction
    - On a patient to determine if an autoimmune response is occurring
  - *Indirect Coombs Test:* This test identifies antibodies that have not but could attach to the patient's RBCs if the patient's blood is mixed. This test is performed:
    - On the blood transfusion recipient or donor before a transfusion to identify if antibodies exist in their blood

11.3 Blood Cultures

Blood cultures are used to assess:

- Existence of bacteria or fungi in blood
- Endocarditis
- Medication that will kill the microorganism
- Cause of unexplained fever
- Effect of treatment for a microorganism infection

Understanding Blood Cultures

Blood can be infected by bacteria or fungi. A blood culture identifies the bacteria or fungi by allowing the microorganism to grow in a controlled environment and then examining the microorganism under a microscope.

The health care provider typically orders a sensitivity test along with the blood culture. The sensitivity test identifies medication that kills the microorganism.

11.4 Mononucleosis Tests

Mononucleosis tests are used to assess for infectious mononucleosis.

Understanding Mononucleosis Tests

The Epstein-Barr virus causes mononucleosis. Mononucleosis tests identify antibodies for the Epstein-Barr virus in the blood sample. There are two kinds of mononucleosis tests:

1. **Monospot:** This test identifies heterophil antibodies that form between 2 weeks and 9 weeks after the patient becomes infected.
2. **EBV Antibody:** This test is ordered when the patient shows symptoms of mononucleosis and the monospot test is negative.

11.5 *Helicobacter pylori* Tests

Helicobacter pylori tests are used to assess for the presence and treatment of *H. pylori*.

Understanding *Helicobacter pylori* Tests

Helicobacter pylori are bacteria that infect the stomach and duodenum, and may result in a peptic ulcer. Many patients have *H. pylori,* but few develop peptic ulcer disease. Four tests are used to detect *H. pylori:*

1. ***H. pylori* Blood Antibody:** This test determines if the blood sample has *H. pylori* antibodies.
2. **Urea Breath:** This test determines the presence of *H. pylori* in the stomach.
3. ***H. pylori* Stool Antigen:** This test determines the presence of *H. pylori* antigens in feces.
4. **Stomach Biopsy:** This is the endoscopic removal of the lining of the stomach and small intestine, which are examined for the presence of *H. pylori*.

All tests may produce a false-negative result if the *H. pylori* count is low and undetectable. The stomach biopsy may produce a false-negative result if the sample was not infected. Blood test for *H. pylori* antibodies may give a false-positive result since antibodies are present years after the *H. pylori* infection is resolved.

11.6 Herpes Tests

Herpes tests are used to assess for the presence of and identification of the type of HSV.

Understanding Herpes Tests

Herpes simplex virus causes painful blister-like sores on the skin and mucous membrane of the mouth, vagina, urethra, rectum, nose, and throat. There are two types of HSV:

- **Herpes Simplex Virus Type 1 (HSV-1):** Commonly called a fever blister or cold sore that appears on the lips that is spread by direct contact or indirectly through sharing eating utensils.
- **Herpes Simplex Virus Type 2 (HSV-2):** Commonly called genital herpes, and appears on the penis or vagina and is spread by direct contact.

There are four common tests for HSV:

1. **Herpes Simplex Virus Antibody Test:** This test identifies HSV antibodies in the blood but cannot differentiate between HSV-1 and HSV-2 and can produce a false-negative result since the immune system takes several days to develop sufficient antibodies to be detected by the HSV antibody test.
2. **Polymerase Chain Reaction (PCR) Test:** This test differentiates between HSV-1 and HSV-2 through cell scraping.
3. **Herpes Virus Antigen Detection Test:** This test detects antigens on cells scraped from the HSV sore using a microscope.
4. **Herpes Viral Culture:** This test cultures cells or fluid from an HSV sore to determine if the sore is from HSV-2.

HSV-1 can infect the genitals. HSV-2 can infect the newborn if the mother has HSV-2. HSV-2 can infect the mouth. There is no cure for HSV; however, the HSV can go into remission. Fatigue, stress, or sunlight can cause HSV sores to recur. Varicella zoster is a type of herpes virus that is better known as shingles and chickenpox.

11.7 Lyme Disease Tests

The Lyme disease tests are used to screen for Lyme disease.

Understanding Lyme Disease Tests

The *Borrelia burgdorferi* bacteria is carried by ticks and transmitted by a tick bite. The Lyme disease tests detect *B. burgdorferi* bacteria antibodies in blood. The health care provider will order at least two of three Lyme disease tests:

- **Indirect Fluorescent Antibody (IFA)**
- **Enzyme-Linked Immunosorbent Assay (ELISA):** This is the quickest and most sensitive test for Lyme disease.
- **Western Blot Test:** This test confirms positive IFA and ELISA test results.

The Lyme disease test can produce a false-negative result if performed within 2 months of the tick bite because the patient's immune system may take 2 months to produce a detectable amount of *B. burgdorferi* bacteria antibodies. Likewise, test results can produce a false-positive result because *B. burgdorferi* bacteria antibodies remain in the patient's blood years after the *B. burgdorferi* bacteria were killed.

The health care provider orders Lyme disease tests if the patient has symptoms of Lyme disease or is known to have been exposed to tick bites.

11.8 Rubella Test

The rubella test is used to assess if the patient is immune to the rubella virus or currently or has recently had a rubella virus infection.

Understanding the Rubella Test

Rubella (German measles) is a virus that causes congenital rubella syndrome (CRS) if a pregnant woman is infected with the rubella virus and transmits it to the fetus in the first trimester. Congenital rubella syndrome consists of birth defects and possibly a miscarriage or stillbirth. The rubella test detects rubella virus antibodies in the blood. There are two rubella virus antibodies that are detected:

- **IgM Antibody:** The patient currently has or recently had a rubella virus infection.
- **IgG Antibody:** The patient has immunity against the rubella virus. The rubella virus antibody developed from a previous rubella virus infection or from the rubella virus vaccination.

11.9 Syphilis Tests

Syphilis tests are used to assess if the patient is infected with syphilis and assess the treatment.

Understanding Syphilis Tests

Treponema pallidum is the bacterium that causes syphilis. The syphilis tests identify *T. pallidum* antibodies in a blood sample. There are seven types of syphilis tests:

1. **Venereal Disease Research Laboratory (VDRL):** This test identifies anticardiolipin antibodies that are produced by a patient who has syphilis. Diseases including syphilis cause the production of anticardiolipin antibodies; therefore, this test is used for screening for syphilis and not diagnosing syphilis.
2. **Rapid Plasma Reagin (RPR):** This test is similar to VDRL except antibodies can be detected without the aid of a microscope.

3. **Enzyme-linked Immunosorbent assay (ELISA):** This test identifies *T. pallidum* antibodies and is used for screening for syphilis. An additional test is necessary to diagnose syphilis.
4. **Fluorescent Treponemal Antibody Absorption (FTA-ABS):** This test identifies *T. pallidum* antibodies after the 4th week after the initial infection and is used to confirm other positive test results.
5. ***Treponema pallidum* Particle Agglutination Assay (TPPA):** This test is similar to the FTA-ABS except it is not used to test spinal fluid.
6. **Darkfield Microscopy:** This test identifies the *T. pallidum* bacterium under a darkfield microscope and is used to diagnose the early stage of syphilis.
7. **Microhemagglutination assay (MHA-TP):** This test is similar to TPPA.

A positive VDRL or RPR test does not mean that the patient has syphilis. Other conditions can cause a positive test result. FTA-ABS, MHA-TP, and TPPA remain positive even after the patient is successfully treated for syphilis. VDRL and RPR tests are negative when treatment for syphilis is successful. A negative result does not rule out syphilis, since detectable antibodies can take 4 weeks to develop following the initial infection.

Many syphilis tests can use either a blood sample or a sample of spinal fluid.

Solved Problems

Infection Tests

11.1 Why are antibody tests administered?

Antibody tests are used to assess the underlying causes of autoimmune hemolytic anemia, blood transfusion reaction, or potential reaction, and screen for the Rh factor.

11.2 What are antibodies?

Antibodies are proteins made by the immune system that bind to bacteria, viruses, and other microorganisms to destroy the microorganism. Antibodies can also bind to red blood cells (RBCs), destroying them as well.

11.3 What is a blood transfusion reaction?

A blood transfusion reaction occurs when transfused blood has different antigens on the surface of its RBCs than the patient's RBCs, which causes the immune system to produce antibodies that attack the transfused RBCs.

11.4 What is rhesus factor sensitization?

Rhesus factor sensitization occurs when the Rh antigen is in the fetus's blood (Rh positive), but not the mother's blood (Rh negative). During delivery, the fetus's blood mixes with the mother's blood, causing the mother's immune system to create antibodies against the fetus's RBCs. The mother becomes Rh sensitive. The antibodies can attack the fetus's RBCs in future pregnancies if the fetus is Rh positive. Women with Rh-negative blood are given the Rh immune globulin (RhoGAM), which typically stops Rh sensitivity.

11.5 What is an Rh antibody titer?

Rh antibody titer is the test performed in early pregnancy to determine the mother's blood type and if the mother is Rh negative.

11.6 What is the direct Coombs test?

The direct Coombs test identifies antibodies attached to the patient's RBCs. This test is performed on a newborn whose mother is Rh negative to determine if the antibodies crossed the placenta into the newborn's blood; a patient who received a blood transfusion to determine if there is a transfusion reaction; and a patient to determine if an autoimmune response is occurring.

11.7 What is the indirect Coombs test?

The indirect Coombs test identifies antibodies that have not but could attach to the patient's red blood cells if the patient's blood is mixed. This test is performed on the blood transfusion recipient or donor before the transfusion to identify if antibodies exist in his or her blood.

11.8 Why would a health care provider order a blood culture?

Blood cultures are used to assess the existence of bacteria or fungi in blood, endocarditis, medication that will kill the microorganism; the cause of unexplained fever; and the effect of treatment of a microorganism infection.

11.9 How is a blood culture performed?

Blood can be infected by bacteria or fungi. A blood culture identifies the bacteria or fungi by allowing the microorganism to grow in a controlled environment and then examining the microorganism under a microscope.

11.10 What is a sensitivity test?

A sensitivity test identifies medication that kills a microorganism.

11.11 What is the virus that causes mononucleosis?

The Epstein-Barr virus causes mononucleosis.

11.12 What is the monospot test?

The monospot test identifies heterophil antibodies that form between 2 and 9 weeks after the patient becomes infected.

11.13 When is the Epstien-Barr virus (EBV) antibody test ordered?

The EBV antibody test is ordered when the patient shows symptoms of mononucleosis and the monospot test is negative.

11.14 What is *Helicobacter pylori*?

H. pylori are bacteria that infect the stomach and duodenum, and may result in a peptic ulcer. Many patients have *H. pylori,* but few develop peptic ulcer disease.

11.15 What is the purpose of the urea breath test?

This test determines the presence of *H. pylori* in the stomach.

11.16 What is the *H. pylori* blood antibody test?

This test determines if the blood sample has *H. pylori* antibodies.

11.17 Why would *H. pylori* tests result in a false-positive result?

Blood tests for *H. pylori* antibodies may give a false-positive result since antibodies are present years after an *H. pylori* infection is resolved.

11.18 Why would *H. pylori* tests result in a false-negative result?

All tests may produce a false-negative result if the *H. pylori* count is low and undetectable.

11.19 What is a common term for herpes simplex virus type 1 (HSV-1)?

HSV-1 is commonly called a fever blister or cold sore that appears on the lips; it is spread by direct contact or indirectly through sharing eating utensils.

11.20 What is herpes simplex virus type 2 (HSV-2)?

HSV-2 is commonly called genital herpes; it appears on the penis or vagina and is spread by direct contact.

11.21 What is the purpose of the polymerase chain reaction (PCR) test?

This test differentiates between HSV-1 and HSV-2 in cell scraping.

11.22 What bacteria cause Lyme disease?

The *Borrelia burgdorferi* bacteria cause Lyme disease.

11.23 Why might the Lyme disease test produce a false-negative result?

Lyme disease test results can produce a false-negative result if performed within 2 months of the tick bite because the patient's immune system may take 2 months to produce a detectable amount of *B. burgdorferi* bacteria antibodies.

11.24 When might the health care provider order Lyme disease tests?

The health care provider might order Lyme disease tests if the patient has symptoms of Lyme disease or is known to have been exposed to tick bites.

11.25 What might be concluded if the patient is positive for the IgM antibody?

The patient currently has or recently had a rubella virus infection.

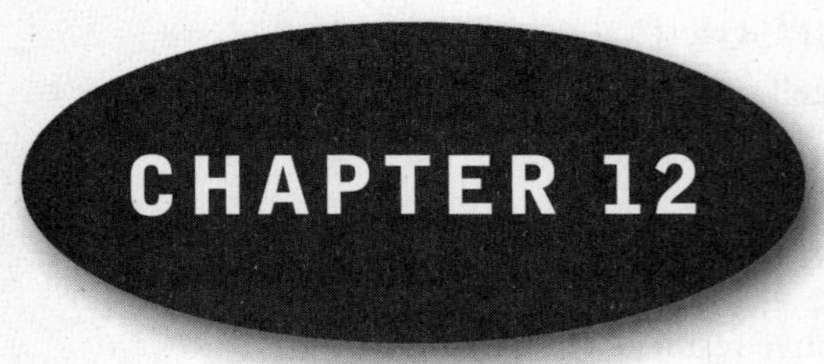

Renal Function Tests

12.1 Definition

Metabolic waste is carried by the blood to the kidneys. The glomerulus in the kidneys acts as a filter to remove waste from the blood, which is collected in a tubule as urine. Metabolic waste such as sodium, potassium, and phosphorus can be reused by the body and are returned to the blood by the kidneys. The remaining waste is excreted as urine.

Renal function is measured in percentages. A person with two healthy kidneys has 100% renal function. Likewise, a person with one healthy kidney and one kidney in total renal failure is considered to have 50% renal function. A person will experience health problems if the person has 25% or less renal function. Dialysis is typically ordered for a patient with <15% renal function.

Renal failure occurs when the glomerulus no longer filters waste from the blood. This can occur suddenly (acute renal failure) in response to illness, medications, accidents, and poisons. It can also happen slowly (chronic kidney disease) from illnesses such as diabetes and high blood pressure. Chronic kidney disease can lead to end-stage renal disease when all or nearly all the renal function is permanently destroyed.

12.2 Blood Urea Nitrogen (BUN) Test

The blood urea nitrogen (BUN) test is used to screen for kidney function and dehydration and assess treatment for kidney disease and kidney dialysis.

Understanding the Blood Urea Nitrogen Test

Ammonia is formed when bacteria in the intestines break down protein. Ammonia is then converted into urea by the liver, which is excreted by the kidney in urine. Urea contains nitrogen. The BUN test measures the level of nitrogen in the blood derived from urea.

The BUN test is typically performed with the creatinine test. The health care provider uses the BUN: creatinine ratio to evaluate the patient's condition.

12.3 Creatinine and Creatinine Clearance Test

The creatinine and creatinine clearance test is used to screen for kidney function and dehydration.

Understanding the Creatinine and Creatinine Clearance Test

Creatine phosphate provides energy to skeletal muscles. After 7 seconds of intense effort, creatine phosphate converts to creatine. Creatine is metabolized into creatinine and is carried in blood to the kidneys for filtering and is excreted in urine. If kidneys are malfunctioning, creatinine levels in the blood increase and creatinine levels in urine decrease. There are three types of creatinine tests:

1. **Blood Creatinine Level:** This test measures the level of creatinine in blood.
2. **Creatinine Clearance:** This test measures creatinine in a 24-hour urine sample and measures the level of creatinine in blood.
3. **Blood Urea Nitrogen: Creatinine Ratio (BUN:creatinine):** This test compares the results of the blood urea test with the blood creatinine level test to assess for dehydration.

A normal blood creatinine level does not rule out kidney disease.

Urea is a by-product of protein metabolism in the liver that is excreted in urine. Fetal kidney function is assessed by testing the level of creatinine in amniotic fluid. The health care provider may order the glomerular filtration rate test to determine kidney function.

Solved Problems

Renal Function Tests

12.1 What is the function of the glomerulus?

The glomerulus in the kidneys acts as a filter to remove waste from the blood.

12.2 What happens to the waste from the blood?

Waste from the blood is collected in a tubule as urine. Metabolic waste such as sodium, potassium, and phosphorus can be reused by the body and are returned to the blood by the kidneys. The remaining waste is excreted as urine.

12.3 How is renal function measured?

Renal function is measured in percentages. A person with two healthy kidneys has 100% renal function. Likewise, a person with one healthy kidney and one kidney in total renal failure is said to have 50% renal function.

12.4 When is dialysis typically ordered?

Dialysis is typically ordered for a patient with <15% renal function.

12.5 When does renal failure occur?

Renal failure occurs when the glomerulus no longer filters waste from the blood.

12.6 What is acute renal failure?

Acute renal failure is the sudden failure of the glomerulus to filter waste from blood in response to illness, medication, accidents, or poisons.

12.7 What is chronic kidney disease?

Chronic kidney disease is the slow failure of the glomerulus to filter waste from blood in response to illness such as diabetes and high blood pressure.

12.8 What is end-stage renal disease?

End-stage renal disease is when all or nearly all the renal function is permanently destroyed.

12.9 What is the purpose of the blood urea nitrogen (BUN) test?

The BUN test is used to screen for kidney function and dehydration and assess treatment for kidney disease and kidney dialysis.

12.10 How does the BUN test work?

The blood urea nitrogen (BUN) test measures the level of nitrogen in the blood derived from urea.

12.11 How is ammonia formed?

Ammonia is formed when bacteria in the intestines break down protein.

12.12 What happens to ammonia in blood?

Ammonia is then converted into urea by the liver.

12.13 What would high-level BUN indicate?

High-level BUN would indicate that there is a high level of ammonia being converted into urea by the liver.

12.14 What is the purpose of the creatinine and creatinine clearance test?

The creatinine and creatinine clearance test is used to screen for kidney function and dehydration.

12.15 What is the purpose of creatine phosphate?

Creatine phosphate provides energy to skeletal muscles.

12.16 What is creatine?

After 7 seconds of intense effort of using skeletal muscles, creatine phosphate converts to creatine.

12.17 What is creatinine?

Creatine is metabolized into creatinine.

12.18 What happens to creatinine?

Creatinine is carried in blood to the kidneys for filtering and is excreted in urine.

12.19 What happens to creatinine if the kidneys malfunction?

If kidneys are malfunctioning, creatinine levels in the blood increase and creatinine levels in urine decrease.

12.20 What is the blood creatinine level test?

The blood creatinine level test measures the level of creatinine in blood.

12.21 What is the creatinine clearance test?

The creatinine clearance test measures creatinine in a 24-hour urine sample and measures the level of creatinine in blood.

12.22 What is the BUN:creatinine ratio?

The BUN:creatinine test compares the results of the blood urea test with the blood creatinine level test to assess for dehydration.

12.23 Does a normal blood creatinine level rule out kidney disease?

No. The level of creatinine may not have as yet reached abnormal levels.

12.24 How is fetal kidney function assessed?

Fetal kidney function is assessed by testing the level of creatinine in amniotic fluid.

12.25 What other test might the health care provider order to determine kidney function?

The health care provider might order the glomerular filtration rate test to determine kidney function.

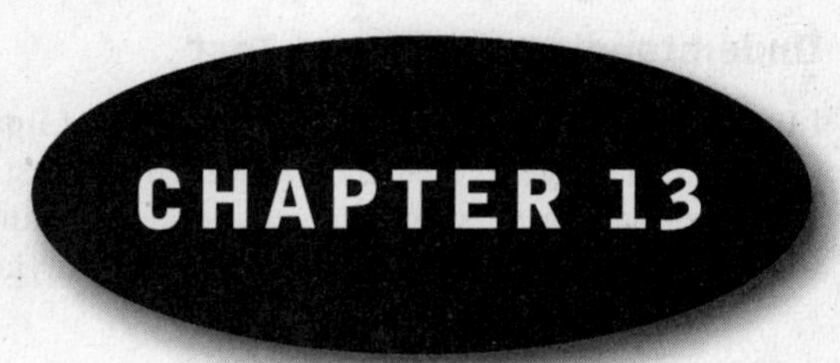

Pancreas and Lipid Metabolism Tests

13.1 Definition

The pancreas produces insulin and glucagon along with digestive enzymes that are used by the small intestine to break down carbohydrates, protein, and fat. Health providers administer pancreatic tests to determine pancreatic function.

Lipids are compounds used to store energy and develop cell membranes, and are elements of vitamins and hormones. Lipids combine with protein to form lipoprotein. Common lipoproteins in the body are cholesterol and triglycerides.

Cholesterol is released into the bloodstream mostly by the liver and other organs, although some cholesterol is ingested in food. Two types of cholesterol are high density lipoprotein (HDL) and low density lipoprotein (LDL).

There is a balance between LDL and HDL. LDL is distributed to cells throughout the body by the bloodstream. Excess LDL is removed by HDL from the blood and transported to the liver, where LDL is metabolized into bile acids and excreted from the body. An imbalance occurs when there is too much LDL in the blood, leading to accumulation of LDL on the artery walls and causing a narrowing of the arteries that leads to a blockage.

Health care providers order lipid metabolism tests to determine the level of lipids in the patient's bloodstream.

13.2 Amylase Test

The amylase test is used to screen for pancreatic disease, pancreatitis, and inflammation of the salivary glands, and assess treatment for pancreatic and salivary gland disease.

Understanding the Amylase Test

Amylase is an enzyme that breaks down starch into sugar. Amylase is produced by the salivary glands and pancreas. The amylase test measures the amount of amylase in blood. There is normally a low level of amylase in blood unless the salivary glands or pancreas is blocked or damaged.

13.3 Lipase Test

The lipase test is used to screen for pancreatic disease, pancreatitis, and cystic fibrosis, and assess treatment for pancreatitis and cystic fibrosis.

Understanding the Lipase Test

Lipase is an enzyme in the pancreas. Levels of lipase in the blood increase when the pancreatic duct is blocked or there is damage to the pancreas. The lipase test measures the level of lipase in blood.

The lipase test does not diagnose pancreatic disorder. A high level of lipase in blood requires additional testing. The health care provider may order the amylase test at the same time as the lipase test.

13.4 Cholesterol and Triglycerides Tests

The cholesterol and triglycerides tests are used to screen for the risk of cardiac disease, assess the underlying cause of yellow fatty deposits in the skin called xanthomas, and assess the treatment for lipid disorder.

Understanding the Cholesterol and Triglycerides Tests

Cholesterol is produced in the liver and used for cell growth and hormone production. Cholesterol attaches to a protein in the blood forming a lipoprotein. Excess cholesterol in the blood forms plaque on the side of blood vessels that can lead to cardiovascular disorders. The cholesterol and triglycerides tests profile the lipoprotein to measure components of cholesterol. These components are:

- **Total Cholesterol:** Total cholesterol is the total amount of LDL and HDL in the blood sample.
- **Low Density Lipoprotein (LDL):** LDL transport lipids from the liver. High levels of LDL increase the risk of cardiovascular disorders.
- **Very Low Density Lipoprotein (VLDL):** VLDL distributes triglycerides that are produced in the liver. High levels of VLDL increase the risk of cardiovascular disorders.
- **High Density Lipoprotein (HDL):** HDL binds with lipids in the blood, returning lipids to the liver, where lipids are metabolized. High levels of HDL decrease the risk of cardiovascular disorders.
- **Triglycerides:** Triglycerides are stored lipids. High levels of triglycerides and high levels of LDL increase the risk of cardiovascular disorders.

Solved Problems

Pancreas and Lipid Metabolism Tests

13.1 What is the function of digestive enzymes produced by the pancreas?

The pancreas produces insulin and glucagon along with digestive enzymes that are used by the small intestine to break down carbohydrates, protein, and fat.

13.2 What are lipids?

Lipids are compounds used to store energy and develop cell membranes, and are elements of vitamins and hormones.

13.3 What is a lipoprotein?

Lipids combine with protein to form a lipoprotein.

13.4 What are common lipoproteins in the body?

Common lipoproteins in the body are cholesterol and triglycerides.

13.5 What releases cholesterol into the bloodstream?

Cholesterol is released into the bloodstream mostly by the liver.

13.6 What are two types of cholesterol in the body?

Two types of cholesterol in the body are high density lipoprotein (HDL) and low density lipoprotein (LDL).

13.7 What is the function of low density lipoprotein (LDL)?

LDL is distributed to cells throughout the body by the bloodstream, where it is used as stored energy and used to develop cell membranes.

13.8 What is the function of high density lipoprotein (HDL)?

Excess LDL is removed by HDL from the blood and transported to the liver.

13.9 What happens to excess LDL?

LDL is metabolized into bile acids by the liver and excreted from the body.

13.10 What happens when there is too much LDL?

An imbalance occurs when too much LDL is in the blood, leading to accumulation of LDL on the artery walls, causing a narrowing of the arteries, and leading to a blockage.

13.11 What is the purpose of the amylase test?

The amylase test is used to screen for pancreatic disease, pancreatitis, and inflammation of the salivary glands, and assessment of treatment for pancreatic and salivary gland disease.

13.12 What is amylase?

Amylase is an enzyme that breaks down starch into sugar.

13.13 Where is amylase produced?

Amylase is produced by the salivary glands and the pancreas.

13.14 What does a low level of amylase in blood indicate?

A low level of amylase in blood is normal.

13.15 What might a high level of amylase in blood indicate?

A high level of amylase in blood indicates that the salivary glands or pancreas are blocked or damaged.

13.16 What is the purpose of the lipase test?

The lipase test is used to screen for pancreatic disease, pancreatitis, and cystic fibrosis, and assess treatment for pancreatitis and cystic fibrosis.

13.17 What is lipase?

Lipase is an enzyme in the pancreas.

13.18 What does a low level of lipase in blood indicate?

A low level of lipase in blood is normal.

13.19 What does a high level of lipase in blood indicate?

A high level of lipase in blood indicates that the pancreatic duct is blocked or there is damage to the pancreas.

13.20 Is the lipase test used to diagnose pancreatic disorders?

No. A high level of lipase in blood requires the health care provider to order additional tests.

13.21 What is the purpose of the cholesterol and triglycerides tests?

The cholesterol and triglycerides tests are used to screen for the risk of cardiac disease, assess the underlying cause of yellow fatty deposits in the skin called xanthomas, and assess the treatment for lipid disorder.

13.22 What is the purpose of the total cholesterol test?

To measure the total amount of LDL and HDL in the blood sample.

13.23 What is the purpose of the low density lipoprotein (LDL) test?

LDL transports lipids from the liver. High levels of LDL increase the risk of cardiovascular disorders.

13.24 What is the purpose of the very low density lipoprotein (VLDL) test?

VLDL distributes triglycerides that are produced in the liver. High levels of VLDL increase the risk of cardiovascular disorders.

13.25 What is the purpose of the high density lipoprotein (HDL) test?

HDL binds with lipids in the blood, returning lipids to the liver where lipids are metabolized. High levels of HDL decrease the risk of cardiovascular disorders.

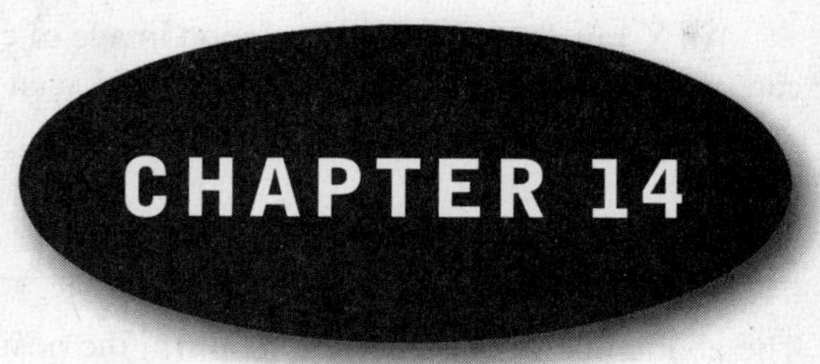

Diagnostic Imaging Tests

14.1 Definition

Diagnostic imaging tests enable the health care provider to view inside the patient's body without opening the skin. Commonly used diagnostic imaging tests are:

- **X-Rays:** X-rays are based on the principle that the X-ray is absorbed by dense objects and will pass through lesser dense objects. Dense objects such as bone appear white on the X-ray file. Less-dense matter such as air appears black, and fluid and fat appear as a lighter shade of gray. X-rays remain a cost-effective way to identify many common disorders.
- **Computed Tomography (CT) Scan:** A computed tomography (CT) scan makes detailed images of structures (with or without contrast medium) within the body using a doughnut-shaped X-ray machine. While the patient lies within the scanner, an X-ray beam rotates around the patient, creating an image that represents a thin slice of the patient.
- **Ultrasound Scan:** An ultrasound scan creates an image of organs and structures inside the body using sound waves. High-frequency sound waves are transmitted by a transducer that is placed on the patient's skin. Sound waves penetrate the skin, bounce off organs and structures in the patient's body, and are detected by the transducer.
- **Magnetic Resonance Imaging (MRI):** A closed magnetic resonance imaging (MRI) uses pulsating radio waves in a magnetic field to produce an image of inside the patient's body. The patient lies on his back on a table. A coil is placed around the area of the patient that is being scanned and a belt is placed around the patient to detect breathing. The table moves into the magnetic field and the belt triggers the MRI scan so that breathing does not interfere with capturing the image. An open MRI does not require that the patient be placed into a machine.
- **Positron Emission Tomography (PET) Scan:** A positron emission tomography (PET) scan is a nuclear medicine test that creates a roadmap of blood flow in the patient's body, enabling the health care provider to visualize abnormal blood flow to the patient's tissues and organs.

14.2 How an X-Ray Is Taken

The patient is positioned between the X-ray gun and a piece of photographic film. The X-ray machine focuses the X-ray beam at the area of the patient's body that is being examined. A portion of the X-ray beam passes through the patient's body, striking the photographic film and leaving a black area on the photographic film. Another portion of the X-ray beam is absorbed by bone and other dense tissue in the patient's body that appear as shades of gray on the photographic film depending on the density of the tissue. Areas that are not being X-rayed are protected by a lead apron where possible to prevent X-rays from reaching those areas.

An X-ray does not provide a good image of cartilage, ligaments, tendons, and other soft tissues. The health care provider will likely order a CT or MRI scan to examine soft tissue.

14.3 Abdominal X-Ray

The abdominal X-ray is used to confirm the position of the nasogastric tube, nephrostomy tube, V-P shunt, or dialysis catheter, and locate an ingested foreign body. An abdominal X-ray is used to assess:

- Underlying cause of abdominal or flank pain
- Underlying cause of vomiting and nausea
- Intestinal blockage
- Perforation in the intestine or stomach

Understanding the Abdominal X-Ray

An abdominal X-ray shows the position, size, and shape of the stomach, diaphragm, liver, spleen, and large and small intestines.

Ovaries are not protected with a lead apron during the X-ray because they are located at the site of the X-ray. An abdominal X-ray cannot detect ulcers or bleeding.

The health care provider may also order a CT scan, ultrasound, or IV pyelograph. A KUB X-ray is an abdominal X-ray that examines the kidneys, uterus, and bladder.

14.4 Extremity X-Ray

The extremity X-ray is used to assess:

- Fracture
- Dislocation
- Tumors
- Deformities/degeneration
- Fluid around joints
- Growths
- Underlying cause of pain in an extremity
- Alignment following treatment
- Infection
- Foreign objects

Understanding the Extremity X-Ray

An extremity X-ray shows damage to hands, wrists, arms, feet, ankles, knees, hips, or legs. The health care provider may not order an X-ray if the results of the X-ray would not alter treatment of the disorder. The health care provider may order a bone scan, CT scan, or MRI if the X-ray does not reveal a disorder.

14.5 Spinal X-Ray

The spinal X-ray is used to assess:

- Fracture
- Dislocation

- Tumors
- Deformities/degeneration
- Curvature of the spine
- Bone spurs
- Underlying cause of weakness, pain, or numbness
- Alignment following treatment

Understanding the Spinal X-Ray

The spine consists of 33 vertebrae, nearly all separated by a disk that absorbs shock related to movement. There are four types of spinal X-rays:

1. **Cervical Spine:** There are seven vertebrae in the cervical area of the spine.
2. **Thoracic Spine:** There are 12 vertebrae in the thoracic area of the spine.
3. **Lumbosacral Spine:** There are five vertebrae in the lumbar area of the spine and five vertebrae in the sacrum area.
4. **Sacrum/Coccyx:** There are five vertebrae in the sacrum area and four vertebrae in the coccyx area.

Strained back muscles or ligaments are not visible on an X-ray. A disk is cartilage.

14.6 Mammogram

The mammogram is used to assess the underlying cause of breast discomfort and to assess if the patient has cysts, solid masses, or calcification in the breast.

Understanding the Mammogram

A mammogram is an X-ray that detects palpable and nonpalpable cysts or masses in the breast, and is used to screen for signs of breast cancer. Suspicious masses are biopsied to determine if the mass is cancerous.

Caution: A mammogram is not normally performed if the patient is pregnant. If the mammogram must be performed, a lead apron is placed over the patient's abdomen.

A mammogram can be performed on a patient who has had breast implants. A mammogram is not performed if the patient is breast-feeding. A breast ultrasound determines if a mass is a cyst or solid mass. A digital mammogram is considered to have the same accuracy as an X-ray mammogram. The health care provider may order the breast cancer (BRCA) gene test if there is a pattern of breast cancer in the patient's family.

The health care provider must provide the patient with the original mammogram images if requested.

14.7 Chest X-Ray

The chest X-ray is used to identify foreign objects in the airway and esophagus, and assess for:

- Pulmonary disease or disorders
- Underlying cause of chest pain or respiratory and cardiac problems
- Chest injury
- Positioning of a medical device

Understanding the Chest X-Ray

A chest X-ray shows the position, size, and shape of the collar bone, breast bone, heart, airway, lungs, thoracic spine, ribs, lymph nodes, and blood vessels. The health care provider may also order an echocardiography, ultrasound, MRI, or CT scan.

14.8 Dental X-Ray

The dental X-ray is used to assess for:

- Cysts, tumors, or abscesses
- Underlying cause of mouth and sinus pain
- Health of teeth
- Position of teeth
- Abnormal structures in the mouth and jaw

Understanding the Dental X-Ray

Dental X-rays are used to assess the condition of the patient's jaw, mouth, and teeth. There are four types of dental X-rays:

1. **Panoramic (orthopantogram):** This type assesses the temporomandibular joints, the jaw, sinuses, teeth, and nasal area for tumors, fractures, cysts, and impacted teeth, but not cavities.
2. **Occlusal:** This type assesses the palate and lower portions of the mouth for fractures, cleft palate, abscesses, tumors, cysts, and immature teeth.
3. **Bitewing:** This type is a single view of the upper and lower back teeth, and is used to assess the formation of teeth, bone loss, infection, and tooth decay.
4. **Periapical:** This type is a view of a tooth, and is used to assess abscesses, tumors, cysts, and the overall status of the patient's teeth.

14.9 Facial X-Ray

The facial X-ray is used to assess:

- Cysts, tumors, or abscesses
- Underlying cause of sinus pain
- Fractures
- Foreign objects

Understanding the Facial X-Ray

A facial X-ray is used to assess facial bones, sinuses, and the orbital cavity. The health care provider may also order a CT scan.

14.10 Skull X-Ray

The skull X-ray is used to assess:

- Cysts, tumors, or abscesses
- Underlying cause of sinus pain
- Fractures
- Foreign objects

Understanding the Skull X-Ray

A skull X-ray is used to assess the skull and sinuses. The health care provider may also order a CT scan.

14.11 How a Computed Tomography (CT) Scan Is Taken

A computed tomography (CT) scan makes detailed images of structures within the body using a doughnut-shaped X-ray machine. While the patient lies within the scanner, an X-ray beam rotates around the patient, creating an image that represents a thin slice of the patient. Each rotation takes less than a second.

All slices are stored on a computer. The computer is used to reassemble slices of the patient, enabling the health care provider to identify any abnormalities. Typically, the health care provider will print the image of any slice that indicates an abnormality, which is then saved with the patient's chart.

The patient may be administered contrast material such as iodine dye. The contrast material makes structures within the patient's body stand out on the computer by differentiating white, black, and shades of gray. Contrast material is administered intravenously or into joints or cavities of the body. The patient may also be asked to ingest other kinds of contrast material.

A CT scan may be used for staging cancer to assess if the cancer has spread to other sites in the body. A CT scan is also used to identify masses or tumors as well as fluid and the infection process. CT scans guide the health care provider when performing a procedure such as a biopsy.

14.12 Full Body CT Scan

The full body CT scan is used to assess:

- Growths
- Obstructions
- Inflammation or infection
- Foreign objects
- Bleeding
- Fluid collection
- Pulmonary embolism

Understanding the Full Body CT Scan

A full body CT scan creates an image of the patient's entire body. A health care provider orders a full body CT scan if it is suspected that the patient may have disorders throughout the body and the health care provider is unable to narrow the disorder to specific areas of the body. This situation may occur if the patient is involved in a severe motor vehicle accident.

Typically, a health care provider orders a CT scan for a specific part of the body rather than ordering a full body scan. A full CT scan is time consuming and usually provides more than enough information necessary for the health care provider to diagnose the patient's disorder. Some health care providers feel that a full body scan identifies benign growths and other disorders that do not adversely affect the patient and could lead to additional tests and surgery that are unnecessary.

The result of a CT scan is commonly compared to the results of a positron emission tomography (PET) scan to identify cancer.

The health care provider must determine if the patient is allergic to shellfish or iodine. Contrast material may contain iodine and other substances that could cause the patient to have an allergic reaction. In addition, the health care provider should determine if the patient will be administered a sedative to relax the patient during the CT scan. If so, the patient must not drive following the CT scan until the sedative has worn off.

14.13 CT Scan of the Head

The CT scan of the head is used to provide baseline images before surgery and assess:

- Growths
- Obstructions

- Inflammation or infection
- Foreign objects
- Bleeding
- Fluid collection
- Headache
- Vertigo
- Vision problems
- Broken bones
- Results of facial surgery
- Temporomandibular disorder
- Paget's disease
- Stroke
- Reasons for change in level of consciousness

Understanding the CT Scan of the Head

The patient's head is placed into the CT scanner as it takes sliced images of the patient's skull, brain, and other parts of the patient's head. The health care provider may order a perfusion CT to determine the blood supply to areas of the brain. Contrast material is administered IV. Areas of the brain that receive blood are highlighted on the computer image by the contrast material. Areas without blood flow are not highlighted.

14.14 CT Scan of the Spine

The CT scan of the spine is used to assess:

- Growths
- Obstructions
- Narrowing of the spinal canal
- Deformities
- Fractures
- Inflammation and infection
- Bone compression
- Osteoporosis
- Congenital defects

Understanding the CT Scan of the Spine

The CT scan of the spine creates images of the cervical, thoracic, and lumbosacral spine. All 33 vertebrae and disks are pictured along with the cerebrospinal fluid (CSF). During the scan, the CT scanner can be tilted to follow the curvature of the spine. Depending on the purpose of the scan, the health care provider may require that contrast material be administered intrathecally into the spinal canal.

14.15 How an Ultrasound Scan Is Taken

An ultrasound scan creates an image of organs and structures inside the body using sound waves similar in concept to how ship crews are able to identify underwater objects while on the surface of the water. High-frequency sound waves are transmitted by a transducer that is placed on the patient's skin.

Sound waves penetrate the skin, bounce off organs and structures in the patient's body, and are detected by the transducer. Sound waves detected by the transducer are translated into an image that appears on the ultrasound screen. The health care provider can then measure organs and structures that appear on the image to determine any abnormality.

Images can be printed and included in the patient's chart or the images can be stored on a computer. An ultrasound can detect a growth but cannot differentiate between a malignant or benign growth, which is determined by a biopsy. An ultrasound can differentiate between a solid growth and a fluid-filled cyst.

Ultrasound scans are commonly ordered instead of a CT scan or MRI because they are less expensive and, in many situations, give the health care provider sufficient information to assist in reaching a diagnosis.

14.16 Benign Prostatic Hyperplasia (BPH) Ultrasound

The benign prostatic hyperplasia (BPH) ultrasound is used to guide the health care provider when taking a biopsy of the prostate and to assess:

- Size of the prostate
- Urinary retention
- Urinary blockage

Understanding the Benign Prostatic Hyperplasia Ultrasound

Middle-aged men might experience the urgency to void, hesitancy waiting for the urinary stream, or a weak urinary stream. These may be signs of an enlarged prostate that places pressure on the bladder and blocks the urinary stream. Noncancerous enlarged prostate is referred to as benign prostatic hyperplasia or hypertrophy. An ultrasound is used to assist the health care provider to diagnose the condition.

The BPH ultrasound is also used to help guide the health care provider when taking a biopsy of the prostate, which is routnely performed if the patient's prostate-specific antigen (PSA) level is elevated. The health care provider may also evaluate the bladder and kidneys while performing the BPH ultrasound to determine urinary retention and kidney stones that may block urinary flow. The BPH ultrasound cannot determine if urinary flow is blocked by the prostate.

14.17 Transvaginal Ultrasound and Hysterosonogram

Transvaginal ultrasound and hysterosonogram are used to guide the health care provider when removing follicles and to schedule intrauterine insemination. It is also used to assess the:

- Uterus
- Fallopian tubes
- Ovaries
- Endometrial cavity
- Uterine lining
- Ovarian follicle development

Understanding the Transvaginal Ultrasound and Hysterosonogram

When a woman has difficulty conceiving, the health care provider may perform a transvaginal ultrasound or a hysterosonogram, also known as a sonohysterogram. These scans enable the health care provider to assess ovarian follicle development and the endometrium. This assessment may help the health care provider determine when to perform intrauterine insemination.

The transvaginal ultrasound is the preferred method rather than the transabdominal ultrasound for assessing the uterine lining and follicle growth. The transvaginal ultrasound may not display scars or small tumors.

14.18 Testicular Ultrasound

The testicular ultrasound is used to guide the health care provider when performing a testicular biopsy. It is also used to assess the:

- Testicles
- Epididymis
- Vas deferens
- Scrotum
- Spermatic cord
- Hydrocele and spermatocele

Understanding the Testicular Ultrasound

A health care provider may order a testicular ultrasound if the patient shows signs and symptoms of testicular abnormalities or infertility. The testicular ultrasound displays an image of the patient's testicles and scrotum, including the epididymis, which is the coiled tube behind the testicle that collects sperm. The testicular ultrasound also displays an image of the vas deferens, which is the tube that connects the prostate gland to the testicles.

14.19 Abdominal Ultrasound

An abdominal ultrasound is used to guide the health care provider when taking a biopsy or performing a paracentesis. It is also used to assess:

- Liver
- Gallbladder
- Bile ducts
- Spleen
- Pancreas
- Kidneys
- Abdominal aorta

Understanding the Abdominal Ultrasound

An abdominal ultrasound is ordered to view upper abdominal organs and structures. These include the liver, gallbladder, spleen, pancreas, and kidneys. It is also ordered to assist the health care provider in assessing the abdominal aorta, which is the artery located in the back of the chest and abdomen that supplies blood to the legs, abdomen, and organs in the lower portion of the body.

The health care provider may order an ultrasound of specific organs or structures within the abdomen if the abdominal ultrasound shows an abnormal condition in the abdomen.

14.20 Breast Ultrasound

The breast ultrasound is used to guide the health care provider when taking a biopsy or when draining a cyst. It is also used to assess:

- Mass found on palpation or by mammogram
- Breast of a younger woman whose breasts are dense
- Silicone breast implants
- Breast pain

Understanding the Breast Ultrasound

The breast ultrasound creates an image of all areas of the breast, including portions that are near the chest. A mammogram typically does not show images of the breast that are near the chest. A breast ultrasound is sometimes performed on younger women whose breast tissues are dense, preventing details of the breast to appear on a mammogram.

A health care provider frequently orders a breast ultrasound to assess a lump identified by either palpation or a mammogram. The breast ultrasound can distinguish between a solid mass and a cyst. If it is a solid mass, then the health care provider performs a biopsy to determine if the mass is benign or malignant.

A breast ultrasound does not replace an annual mammogram.

14.21 Cranial Ultrasound

The cranial ultrasound is used to assess a brain mass in an adult. For a baby, it is used to assess:

- Why the baby has an abnormally large head
- Encephalitis
- Meningitis
- Hydrocephalus
- Periventricular leukomalacia (PVL)
- Intraventricular hemorrhage (IVH)

Understanding the Cranial Ultrasound

A cranial ultrasound creates images of the brain and ventricles. Since ultrasound cannot penetrate bone, a cranial ultrasound is performed on babies up to 18 months old whose cranium has yet to form. A cranial ultrasound is commonly used in premature newborns to assess complications of the premature birth.

A cranial ultrasound is also performed on adults during brain surgery to visualize any masses in the brain. The ultrasound is able to capture the image because a portion of the patient's cranium is removed during surgery, enabling the ultrasound to penetrate brain tissue.

14.22 Doppler Ultrasound

The Doppler ultrasound is used to map veins for use as grafts and assess for:

- Narrow blood vessels
- Blood clots (deep vein thrombosis)
- Atherosclerosis
- Stroke

Understanding the Doppler Ultrasound

A Doppler ultrasound is used to assess blood flow through blood vessels. There are four types of Doppler ultrasounds:

1. **Continuous Wave:** This test produces a pulsating audible sound reflecting pulsating blood through a blood vessel.
2. **Duplex:** This test produces an image of the blood vessel along with a computer-generated graph indicating the speed and direction of blood flow.
3. **Color:** This test produces an image of the blood vessel with the speed and direction of blood flow represented by colors on the image.

4. **Power:** This test is similar to the color Doppler; however, the power Doppler is five times as sensitive in detecting blood flow.

14.23 Fetal Ultrasound

The fetal ultrasound is used to detect ectopic pregnancy and assess:

- Progress of the pregnancy
- Gestational age of the fetus
- Fetal defects
- Number of fetuses
- Placenta
- Amniotic fluid
- Fetal position
- Cervix

Understanding the Fetal Ultrasound

A fetal ultrasound produces an image (sonogram) of the fetus, placenta, and amniotic fluid during pregnancy. The health care provider orders a fetal ultrasound to determine the size, position, and sex of the fetus, and to identify any abnormalities prior to birth. There are two types of fetal ultrasound tests:

1. **Transabdominal:** The ultrasound transducer is placed on the patient's abdomen.
2. **Transvaginal:** The ultrasound transducer is covered in a latex sheath and inserted into the vagina.

The health care provider must verify that the patient is not allergic to latex if performing a transvaginal ultrasound. A normal fetal ultrasound does not rule out fetal abnormalities or problems with the placenta and amniotic fluid.

14.24 Pelvic Ultrasound

The pelvic ultrasound is used to guide the health care provider when performing a biopsy and is used to assess for:

- Cause of urinary disorders
- Bladder
- Existence of growths
- Pelvic inflammatory disease (PID)
- Placement of an intrauterine device (IUD)
- Size of pelvic organs and structures
- Fetal position
- Cause of infertility

Understanding the Pelvic Ultrasound

A pelvic ultrasound creates images of the bladder, ovaries, uterus, cervix, fallopian tubes, prostate gland, and seminal vesicles. There are three types of pelvic ultrasound tests:

1. **Transabdominal:** The transducer is moved along the abdomen.
2. **Transrectal:** The transducer is inserted in the rectum.
3. **Transvaginal:** The transducer is covered with a latex sheath and inserted in the vagina.

The health care provider must verify that the patient is not allergic to latex before a transrectal or transvaginal ultrasound is performed.

14.25 Thyroid and Parathyroid Ultrasound

The thyroid or parathyroid ultrasound is used to guide the health care provider when performing a biopsy and used to assess for:

- Size of the thyroid gland
- Size of the parathyroid gland
- Growths

Understanding the Thyroid and Parathyroid Ultrasound

The thyroid and parathyroid ultrasound is used to create images of the thyroid and parathyroid glands. The thyroid gland produces thyroxine, which controls the patient's metabolism. The parathyroid gland produces the parathyroid hormone (PTH), which controls the patient's calcium and phosphorus balance in the blood.

The thyroid and parathyroid ultrasound enables the health care provider to assess the size of these glands but not the production of hormones.

14.26 How a Magnetic Resonance Image (MRI) Is Taken

Magnetic resonance imaging (MRI) uses pulsating radio waves in a magnetic field to produce an image of the inside of the patient's body. The patient lies on his or her back on a table. A coil is placed around the area of the patient who is being scanned and a belt is placed around the patient to detect breathing. The table moves into the magnetic field and the belt triggers the MRI scan so that breathing does not interfere with capturing the image. A snapping noise is heard while the MRI scans the patient. The patient may listen to music through headphones to block out the snapping noise.

There are two types of MRI machines: *closed MRI* and *open MRI*. In the closed MRI, the patient's body is entirely enclosed in the machine, whereas in an open MRI only a portion of the patient's body is enclosed.

The health care provider may order that contrast material be administered to the patient prior to the MRI. The contrast material may be ingested or administered intravenously and highlight areas of the body that are being studied. The MRI produces digital images that are displayed on a computer screen and can be stored for further review by the patient's health care team. The MRI creates images that are more detailed than images produced by a CT scan, X-ray, or ultrasound.

No metal objects can be on or inside the patient during an MRI, including credit cards. Information on the credit card might be erased by the MRI magnetic field. An X-ray may be ordered to determine if there is any metal inside the patient before the MRI is administered, especially if the patient was in an accident during which metal fragments might have been embedded throughout the body.

However, dental fillings are usually permitted, although the patient is likely to feel tingling in the mouth during the MRI. The patient may experience skin irritation if the patient has iron pigment tattoos.

14.27 Abdominal MRI

The abdominal MRI is used to guide the health care provider when performing a biopsy and used to assess:

- Size of abdominal organs and structures
- Existence of a growth
- Existence and then identification of a blockage

- Existence of fluid within the abdomen
- Inflammation
- Blood flow

Understanding the Abdominal MRI

An abdominal MRI produces detailed images of organs, structures, and tissues contained within the abdomen. The health care provider may order that the patient be administered contrast material prior to the MRI to highlight parts of the abdomen on the MRI image. This enables the health care provider to identify any subtle abnormalities that may exist in the abdomen.

14.28 Breast MRI

The breast MRI is used to assess:

- Infection
- Existence of a growth
- Inflammation
- Blood flow
- Women who are at a high risk for breast cancer
- Women who normally have dense breast tissue
- Breast cancer treatment
- Breast implants

Understanding the Breast MRI

A breast MRI produces detailed images of the breast that provide more information to the health care provider than a breast ultrasound or traditional mammogram. Health care providers typically order breast MRIs when other tests such as a mammogram indicate an abnormality. If the abnormality is inflammation, a growth, or blood flow to breast tissues, the health care provider may administer contrast material to enhance the image of those areas of the breast.

Women who are positive for the BRCA1 or BRCA2 gene or whose family members developed breast cancer before the age of 50 are considered at high risk for developing breast cancer and may be recommended for annual breast MRIs to detect early signs of breast cancer. The health care provider may also order an annual breast MRI for women who normally have dense breast tissue. An MRI is better suited to examine dense breast tissue than an ultrasound test.

14.29 Head MRI

The head MRI is used to assess:

- Infection
- Existence of a growth
- Inflammation
- Blood flow
- Stroke
- Suspected head injury
- Hydrocephaly

- Multiple sclerosis (MS)
- Alzheimer's disease
- Parkinson's disease
- Huntington's disease

Understanding the Head MRI

An MRI of the head is ordered to produce images of the brain and blood vessels that supply blood to the brain to determine the underlying cause of headache, assess for head injury, or determine if the patient has abnormal blood flow or a disorder that affects the brain. Unlike an ultrasound, the head MRI is a closed procedure and does not require that the patient's skull be opened. There are three types of MRI used to assess the brain:

1. **Magnetic Resonance Spectroscopy:** This test assesses changes in brain chemistry caused by disease.
2. **Magnetic Resonance Angiogram (MRA):** This test assesses the speed, direction, and flow of blood in the brain.
3. **Diffusion-Perfusion Imaging:** This test assesses inflammation, tumors, and stroke, but evaluates the fluid content of the brain.

Health care providers may order an MRI with gadolinium-containing contrast material. Gadolinium can cause nephrogenic fibrosing dermopathy in patients who have kidney failure.

14.30 Knee MRI

The knee MRI is used to assess:

- Knee structures and tissues
- Existence of a growth
- Arthritis
- Tendons, ligaments, cartilage, or meniscus
- If arthroscopy is required

Understanding the Knee MRI

A knee MRI produces detailed images of structures and tissues contained within the knee. This enables the health care provider to identify any abnormalities that may exist in the knee, including damage to tendons, ligaments, cartilage, and fluid. The health care provider may order a knee MRI to assess if the patient requires arthroscopy of the knee.

14.31 Shoulder MRI

The shoulder MRI is used to assess:

- Shoulder structures and tissues
- Existence of a growth
- Arthritis
- Tendons, ligaments, cartilage, bones, or muscles
- Rotator cuff disorders
- If arthroscopy is required

Understanding the Shoulder MRI

The shoulder MRI is ordered to show the health care provider detailed images of inside the shoulder, including ligaments, cartilage, muscles, and bone structure within the shoulder and fluid. These images are more detailed than can be achieved using ultrasound and CT scans, and are commonly ordered to assess shoulder pain that is unexplained by other signs or symptoms.

14.32 Spinal MRI

The spinal MRI is used to assess:

- Spinal structures and tissues
- Ruptured disk
- Sciatica
- Spinal stenosis
- Existence of growths
- Arthritis
- Damaged nerves

Understanding the Spinal MRI

The spinal MRI shows detailed images of the patient's spine. This includes the cervical, thoracic, and lumbosacral spine. The spinal MRI helps the health care provider assess if the patient has spinal disk disorders or spinal stenosis, as well as tumors and arthritis. The health care provider also orders a spinal MRI to assess unexplained spinal pain.

14.33 Positron Emission Tomography (PET) Scan

The positron emission tomography (PET) scan is used to assess:

- Blood flow to organs and tissues
- Metabolic activity or organs
- Stroke and transient ischemic attack (TIA)
- Multiple sclerosis
- Parkinson's and Alzheimer's diseases
- Epilepsy
- Coronary artery disease
- Presence of cancer and to determine if the cancer has metastasized

Understanding the Positive Emission Scan

The positive emission scan is ordered to study blood flow and metabolic activity within a patient's body. Health care providers frequently combine results from the PET scan with CT scan results to obtain a thorough understanding of how well tissues and organs are being infused with blood.

Sometimes a CT scan is performed along with a PET scan. The tracer contains low-level radiation that will rarely lead to tissue damage. The tracer is flushed from the patient's body in 24 hours following the scan. It is rare that a patient will have an allergic reaction to the tracer. The health care provider may order a single photon emission computed tomography (SPECT) scan to determine if a patient with chest pain is at risk for cardiac arrest.

14.34 How a Positron Emission Tomography (PET) Scan Is Taken

A positron emission tomography (PET) scan is a nuclear medicine test that creates a roadmap of blood flow in the patient's body, enabling the health care provider to visualize abnormal blood flow to the patient's tissues and organs.

A radioactive chemical called a tracer and a special camera that detects the tracer inside the patient's body are the keys to a PET scan. The health care provider administers the tracer into the patient's veins prior to the scan. The tracer gives off positrons, which are very small charged particles that can be detected by the PET scan camera. The PET scan camera takes a series of images, each capturing the position of positrons in the body. These images are stored and replayed on a computer screen. These images show the tracer containing blood as the blood makes its way into organs and tissues, giving the health care provider a clear picture of blood flow within the body.

14.35 Bone Mineral Density (BMD) Test

The bone mineral density (BMD) test is ordered to assess for osteoporosis, the progression of osteoporosis, and the impact of long-term corticosteroid treatment.

Understanding the Bone Mineral Density Test

The bone mineral density test measures the density of bone to assess if the patient has osteopenia or osteoporosis. A low bone density might result in increased risk for fracture. There are five ways to measure bone mineral density:

1. **Ultrasound:** This test uses sound waves to determine the density of bone. However, this method does not assess the hip and spine, which are bones that commonly fracture because of low bone mineral density.
2. **Dual-Photo Absorptiometry (DPA):** This method uses a low-dose radioactive tracer to measure bone density in all bones, including the hip and spine.
3. **Quantitative Computed Tomography (QCT):** This method measures the density of the vertebra; however, this is less accurate than the DPA, DEXA, and P-DEXA methods.
4. **Dual-Energy X-Ray Absorptiometry (DEXA):** This method uses two X-ray beams to measure bone density and can measure up to 2% bone loss, making it the most accurate way to measure bone mineral density.
5. **Peripheral Dual-Energy X-Ray Absorptiometry (PDEXA):** This method measures bone density in the arms and legs, but cannot be used to measure the bone density of the hip or spine.

14.36 Bone Scan

A bone scan assesses infection, trauma, and metastasized cancer growth to the bone.

Understanding the Bone Scan

A radioactive tracer is injected in the patient's vein. The tracer is removed from the blood into the bone. A gamma camera takes an image of the tracer as the tracer is absorbed. Lack of absorption indicates bone infarction and possibly cancer. Areas of high absorption might indicate an infection, tumor, or fracture.

Solved Problems

Diagnostic Imaging Tests

14.1 What appears white on an X-ray?

Dense objects such as bone appear white on an X-ray.

14.2 What appears black or a lighter shade of gray on an X-ray?

Less-dense matter such as air appears black and fluid and fat appear as a lighter shade of gray.

14.3 Why are X-rays still taken rather than using more advanced imaging technology?

X-rays remain a cost-effective way to identify many common disorders.

14.4 How does a computed tomography (CT) scan work?

A CT scan makes detailed images of structures within the body using a doughnut-shaped X-ray machine. While the patient lies within the scanner, an X-ray beam rotates around the patient, creating an image that represents a thin slice of the patient.

14.5 How does an ultrasound scan work?

An ultrasound scan creates an image of organs and structures inside the body using sound waves. High-frequency sound waves are transmitted by a transducer that is placed on the patient's skin. Sound waves penetrate the skin, bounce off organs and structures in the patient's body, and are detected by the transducer.

14.6 How does a magnetic resonance imaging (MRI) work?

An MRI uses pulsating radio waves in a magnetic field to produce an image of inside the patient's body. The patient lies on his or her back on a table. A coil is placed around the area of the patient that is being scanned and a belt is placed around the patient to detect breathing. The table moves into the magnetic field and the belt triggers the MRI scan so that breathing does not interfere with capturing the image.

14.7 How does a positron emission tomography (PET) scan work?

A PET scan is a nuclear medicine test that creates a roadmap of blood flow in the patient's body, enabling the health care provider to visualize abnormal blood flow to the patient's tissues and organs.

14.8 Why would a health care provide not order an X-ray?

An X-ray does not provide a good image of cartilage, ligaments, tendons, and other soft tissues; therefore, the health care provider will likely order a CT scan or MRI to examine soft tissue.

14.9 Why might a health care provider not order an extremity X-ray if the patient has an obvious fracture?

The health care provider may not order an X-ray if the results of the X-ray would not alter treatment of the disorder.

14.10 If the patient who is suspected of having a bone disorder is given an X-ray and the X-ray does not reveal the disorder, what might the health care provider do?

The health care provider might order a bone scan, CT scan, or MRI if the X-ray does not reveal a disorder.

14.11 What is a lumbosacral spine X-ray?

A lumbosacral spine X-ray examines the five vertebrae in the lumbar area of the spine and five vertebrae in the sacrum area.

14.12 How would you respond if the patient said that the health care provider ordered an X-ray because she suspects injury to a spinal disk?

Explain that the health care provider probably ordered a different imaging test because a spinal disk is cartilage and cartilage is not visible on an X-ray.

14.13 What is the purpose of a bitewing X-ray?

The bitewing type of X-ray is a single view of the upper and lower back teeth and is used to assess the formation of teeth, bone loss, infection, and tooth decay.

14.14 Why might a patient be administered contrast material before undergoing a CT scan?

The contrast material makes structures within the patient's body standout on the computer by differentiating between white, black, and shades of gray.

14.15 What are the limitations of the ultrasound when assessing growths?

An ultrasound can detect a growth but cannot differentiate between a malignant or benign growth, which is determined by a biopsy. An ultrasound can differentiate between a solid growth and a fluid-filled cyst.

14.16 Why are ultrasounds ordered instead of a CT scan or MRI?

Ultrasound scans are commonly ordered instead of a CT scan or MRI because they are less expensive and in many situations give the health care provider sufficient information to assist to reach a diagnosis.

14.17 What is the purpose of a BPH ultrasound?

The benign prostatic hyperplasia (BPH) ultrasound is used to guide the health care provider when taking a biopsy of the prostate and to assess for the size of the prostate, urinary retention, and a urinary blockage.

14.18 What is a limitation of the BPH ultrasound?

The benign prostatic hyperplasia ultrasound cannot determine if urinary flow is blocked by the prostate.

14.19 What is the preferred method of assessing the uterine lining and follicle growth?

The transvaginal ultrasound is the preferred method for assessing the uterine lining and follicle growth rather than the transabdominal ultrasound.

14.20 What is a common reason that the health care provider orders a breast ultrasound?

A health care provider frequently orders a breast ultrasound to assess a lump identified by either palpation or from a mammogram. The breast ultrasound can distinguish between a solid mass and a cyst.

14.21 What is the purpose of a Doppler ultrasound?

The Doppler ultrasound is used to map veins for use as grafts and to assess narrow blood vessels, and for blood clots (deep vein thrombosis), atherosclerosis, and stroke.

14.22 What is a continuous wave Doppler?

Continuous wave Doppler produces a pulsating audible sound, reflecting pulsating blood through a blood vessel.

14.23 What is the purpose of a color Doppler?

Color Doppler produces an image of the blood vessel with the speed and direction of blood flow represented by colors on the image.

14.24 Why might a health care provider order a fetal ultrasound?

The fetal ultrasound is used to detect ectopic pregnancy and assess progress of the pregnancy, gestational age of the fetus, for fetal defects, the number of fetuses, the placenta, amniotic fluid, the fetal position, and the cervix.

14.25 What is the difference between a closed and open MRI?

In the closed MRI, the patient's body is entirely enclosed in the machine, whereas only a portion of the patient's body is enclosed in an open MRI machine.

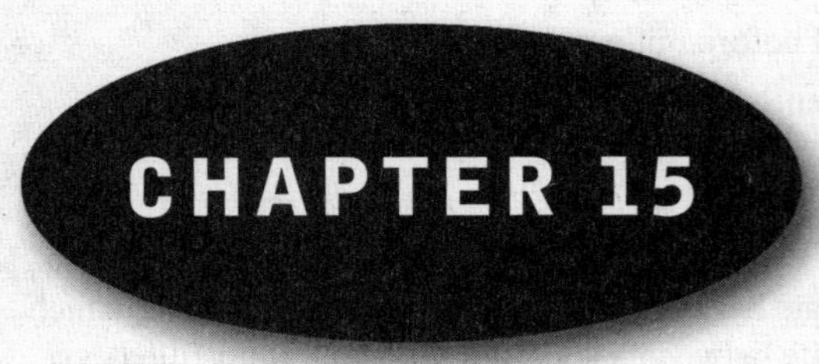

Biopsy

15.1 Definition

When a patient has a growth or unusual fluid buildup in the body, the health care provider will likely order noninvasive tests such as an X-ray, CT, or MRI scan that displays an image of the affected portion of the patient's body.

If the health care provider is unable to diagnose the patient based on signs, symptoms, and images, the health care provider may take a biopsy of the suspicious tissue. In a biopsy, the health care provider removes a small sample of the tissue and sends the sample to a pathologist, who conducts a microscopic study of the tissue to reach a definitive diagnosis. The pathologist determines the type of cells in the sample and whether they are benign or malignant.

Tissue samples are collected by scraping cells on the cervix for a pap smear or the insertion of a large-bore needle to remove a larger number of cells called a core sample (e.g., larger sections of tissue can be removed for study using surgical techniques).

A negative biopsy result does not guarantee that the patient is free of cancer. It simply means that no cancer cells were found in the sample tissue.

15.2 Lung Biopsy

The lung biopsy is used to assess growths identified on an X-ray, CT, or MRI scan, and is used to diagnose lung cancer and other lung disorders.

Understanding the Lung Biopsy

A lung biopsy is the sampling of lung tissue that appears suspicious on a chest X-ray or CT scan. Typically, a health care provider orders a lung biopsy when signs and symptoms point to lung cancer, pulmonary fibrosis, sarcoidosis, or other lung diseases. There are four methods used to take a lung biopsy:

1. **Needle:** With the guidance of an ultrasound or CT scan, the health care provider inserts a long needle through the chest wall and into the lung to remove tissue.
2. **Bronchoscope:** A bronchoscope is inserted into the patient's airway by the health care provider and a tissue sample is removed from the bronchi.
3. **Video-assisted Thoracoscopic Surgery (VATS):** The health care provider makes an incision into the patient's chest and inserts a thoracoscope into the incision to remove lung tissue.
4. **Open:** The health care provider makes an incision between the patient's ribs and into the lungs to remove lung tissue. This is commonly performed if a large tissue sample is being examined or if less intrusive biopsy methods are unsuccessful.

15.3 Percutaneous Kidney Biopsy

The percutaneous kidney biopsy is used to assess growths identified on a CT scan or ultrasound and is used to diagnose kidney cancer and other kidney disorders.

Understanding the Percutaneous Kidney Biopsy

A kidney biopsy is the sampling of kidney tissue when urinalysis indicates protein or blood in the urine or a CT or ultrasound scan shows a growth in or on the kidney. A kidney biopsy is sometimes performed to assess the progress of disease that affects the kidneys.

15.4 Liver Biopsy

The liver biopsy is used to assess growths identified on a CT scan or ultrasound and is used to diagnose liver cancer and other liver disorders. It is also used to identify the underlying cause of jaundice or abnormal liver enzyme test results. A liver biopsy is also used to assess the effect of medication on the liver and assess treatment for liver disorders.

Understanding the Liver Biopsy

A liver biopsy is the sampling of liver tissue. The sample is taken by inserting a needle between two right lower ribs. A liver biopsy is typically ordered when a CT or ultrasound scan identifies a growth or unexpected shape of the liver.

15.5 Lymph Node Biopsy

The lymph node biopsy is used to identify an abnormality that is causing the lymph node to swell.

Understanding the Lymph Node Biopsy

All fluids in the body, including abnormal cells such as cancer cells, are filtered by lymph nodes located throughout the body. Lymph nodes might increase in size when fluids are trapped by the filter, giving the appearance of swollen lymph nodes, which may be a sign that something is wrong with the patient. A health care provider may take a biopsy of one or more lymph nodes to identify the antigen.

15.6 Sentinel Lymph Node Biopsy

The sentinel lymph node biopsy is used to assess the spread of cancer cells.

Understanding the Sentinel Lymph Node Biopsy

A sentinel lymph node biopsy removes tissue samples from one or more lymph nodes to determine if cancer cells have spread from the site of the cancer. The sentinel node is the node most likely to indicate cancer cells may have spread from the primary cancer site. If the sentinel lymph node biopsy is positive, then the health care provider will likely order a lymph node dissection, which is the removal of the entire lymph node.

15.7 Testicular Biopsy

The testicular biopsy is used to assess if the patient is infertile.

Understanding the Testicular Biopsy

The testicular biopsy removes tissue samples from one or both testicles to determine if the patient is infertile. A testicular biopsy is not performed to determine if the patient has testicular cancer. An orchiectomy, which is a surgical procedure, is performed to diagnose testicular cancer.

15.8 Thyroid Biopsy

The thyroid biopsy is used to assess an enlarged thyroid gland (goiter) or assess a growth on the thyroid gland.

Understanding the Thyroid Biopsy

The thyroid biopsy removes tissue samples of the thyroid gland to determine if the patient has thyroid cancer or other thyroid disorders. There are two types of thyroid biopsies:

1. **Fine-Needle:** A needle is inserted through the skin into the thyroid gland to retrieve sample cells.
2. **Open:** An incision is made through the skin, making the thyroid gland visible to the health care provider as tissue samples are retrieved. The open biopsy is performed under general anesthesia.

15.9 Prostate Biopsy

The prostate biopsy is used to assess an enlarged prostate gland or to assess a growth on the prostate gland.

Understanding the Prostate Biopsy

A prostate biopsy removes tissue samples of the prostate gland to determine if the patient has prostate cancer. There are three types of prostate biopsies:

1. **Transrectal:** A needle is inserted through the rectum to remove samples of prostate tissue.
2. **Transurethral:** A needle is inserted through the urethra to remove samples of prostate tissue.
3. **Transperineal:** A needle is inserted in the skin between the anus and scrotum to remove samples of prostate tissue.

15.10 Skin Biopsy

The skin biopsy is used to assess changes in the skin.

Understanding the Skin Biopsy

A skin biopsy removes tissue samples of the skin to identify skin lesions that have changed in color, size, and appearance. There are four common skin biopsies:

1. **Shave:** A sample of the skin lesion is shaved using a scalpel.
2. **Excision:** The entire skin lesion is removed from the patient.
3. **Punch:** A circular sample of the skin lesion is removed using a punch.
4. **Incision:** A piece of the skin lesion is removed from the patient.

Solved Problems

Biopsy

15.1 What is a biopsy?

The health care provider removes a small sample of the tissue and sends the sample to a pathologist, who conducts a microscopic study of the tissue to reach a definitive diagnosis.

15.2 What is meant by a negative biopsy result?

No cancer cells were found in the sample tissue.

15.3 Does a negative biopsy results guarantee that the patient is free of cancer?

No. It means that no cancer cells were found in the sample tissue.

15.4 What is the purpose of a lung biopsy?

The lung biopsy is used to assess growths identified on an X-ray, CT, or MRI scan, and is used to diagnose lung cancer and other lung disorders.

15.5 What is a needle biopsy?

With the guidance of an ultrasound or CT scan, the health care provider inserts a long needle through the chest wall and into the lung to remove tissue.

15.6 What is a bronchoscope biopsy?

A bronchoscope is inserted into the patient's airway by the health care provider and a tissue sample is removed from the bronchi.

15.7 What is video-assisted thoracoscopic surgery (VATS)?

Video-assisted thoracoscopic surgery (VATS) occurs when the health care provider makes an incision into the patient's chest and inserts a thorascope into the incision to remove lung tissue.

15.8 What is an open biopsy?

The health care provider makes an incision between the patient's ribs and into the lungs to remove lung tissue. This is commonly performed if a large tissue sample is being examined or less intrusive biopsy methods are unsuccessful.

15.9 What is the purpose of a percutaneous kidney biopsy?

The percutaneous kidney biopsy is used to assess growths identified on a CT scan or ultrasound and is used to diagnose kidney cancer and other kidney disorders.

15.10 When might a percutaneous kidney biopsy be ordered?

A kidney biopsy is the sampling of kidney tissue when urinalysis indicates protein or blood in the urine or a CT or ultrasound scan shows a growth in or on the kidney.

15.11 What is the purpose of a liver biopsy?

The liver biopsy is used to assess growths identified on a CT scan or ultrasound and is used to diagnose liver cancer and other liver disorders. It is also used to identify the underlying cause of jaundice or abnormal liver enzyme test results. A liver biopsy is also used to assess the effect of medication on the liver and assess treatment for liver disorder.

15.12 When might a liver biopsy be ordered?

A liver biopsy is typically ordered when a CT or ultrasound scan identifies a growth or unexpected shape of the liver.

15.13 How is a liver biopsy performed?

A liver biopsy is the sampling of liver tissue. The sample is taken by inserting a needle between two right lower ribs.

15.14 Why might a lymph node biopsy be ordered?

All fluids in the body, including abnormal cells such as cancer cells, are filtered by lymph nodes located throughout the body. Lymph nodes might increase in size when fluids are trapped by the filter, giving the appearance of swollen lymph nodes, which may be a sign that something is wrong with the patient. A health care provider may take a biopsy of one or more lymph nodes to identify the antigen.

15.15 What is the purpose of a sentinel lymph node?

The sentinel lymph node biopsy is used to assess the spread of cancer cells.

15.16 What is a sentinel lymph node?

The sentinel lymph node is the node most likely to indicate cancer cells may have spread from the primary cancer site.

15.17 What might be ordered if the sentinel lymph node biopsy is positive?

If the sentinel lymph node biopsy is positive, then the health care provider will likely order a lymph node dissection, which is the removal of the entire lymph node.

15.18 Why might a health care provider order a testicular biopsy?

The testicular biopsy is used to assess if the patient is infertile.

15.19 Is a testicular biopsy used to diagnose testicular cancer?

A testicular biopsy is not performed to determine if the patient has testicular cancer. An orchiectomy, which is a surgical procedure, is performed to diagnose testicular cancer.

15.20 What is a transrectal biopsy?

A transrectal biopsyoccurs when a needle is inserted through the rectum to remove samples of prostate tissue.

15.21 What is a transurethral biopsy?

A transurethral biopsy occurs when a needle is inserted through the urethra to remove samples of prostate tissue.

15.22 What is a transperineal biopsy?

A transperineal biopsy occurs when a needle is inserted in the skin between the anus and scrotum to remove samples of prostate tissue.

15.23 What is an excision biopsy?

An excision biopsy occurs when the entire skin lesion is removed from the patient.

15.24 What is a punch biopsy?

A punch biopsy occurs when a circular sample of the skin lesion is removed using a punch.

15.25 What is an incision biopsy?

An incision biopsy occurs when a piece of the skin lesion is removed from the patient.

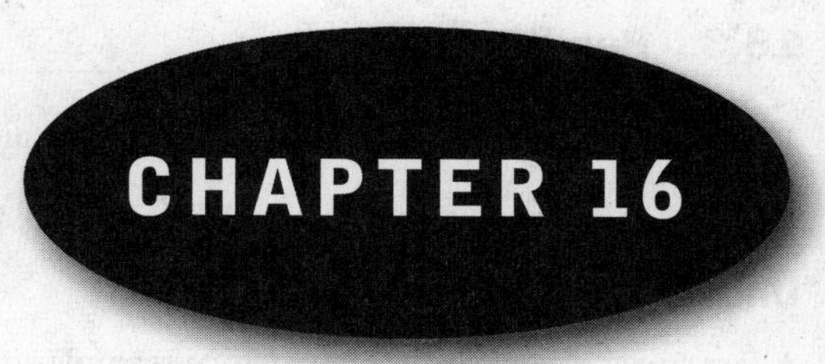

Female Tests

16.1 Definition

Female patients routinely undergo breast and cervical examinations for signs of cysts, growths, abnormal tissue, structural abnormalities, and infection. In this chapter, you will learn about tests and procedures that are performed to test for disorders and their repair.

When a mammogram reveals a suspicious growth, the health care provider usually orders a breast ultrasound to closely examine the growth and then possibly orders a breast biopsy. If the tissue sample is deemed cancerous via the breast biopsy results, the health care provider may perform a mastectomy. A mastectomy may be performed even if there are no signs of breast cancer. Reasons for performing a mastectomy without empirical evidence of cancer are explored in this chapter. The patient may decide to have her breasts altered for therapeutic or cosmetic reasons. You will learn about procedures that augment, reduce, and lift the breast in this chapter.

There are a number of tests used to examine the patient's vulva, vagina, cervix, uterus, and fallopian tubes. Many of these tests enable the health care provider to take a tissue sample or perform a biopsy on abnormal tissue. If the tissue sample is identified to be cancerous, the cancerous organ is removed. You will learn about these tests and procedures in this chapter.

16.2 Breast Cancer Gene (BRCA) Test

The breast cancer gene (BRCA) test is used to assess the patient's chances of developing breast or ovarian cancer.

Understanding the Breast Cancer Gene Test

Scientists have discovered two genes called the breast cancer genes (BRCA1, BRCA2) that are associated with breast and ovarian cancer if mutated. A patient who carries this mutated gene and has a family history of breast or ovarian cancer may have a higher than normal chance of developing breast or ovarian cancer. However, the patient also has a chance of not developing these cancers. The presence of the breast cancer gene does not mean that the patient will develop breast or ovarian cancer. The breast cancer gene test determines if the patient's BRCA1 and BRCA2 genes are mutated. If so, some patients may decide to have a mastectomy and/or oophorectomy to prevent these cancers from developing. Patients who test positive may also be advised to take tamoxifen to inhibit this gene.

Male patients who have a family history of breast and prostate cancer may also have this gene. These patients can also develop breast and prostate cancer.

16.3 Pap Smear

The Pap smear is used to assess cervical tissue and identify abnormal cervical tissues that might be cancerous or precancerous in nature.

Understanding the Pap Smear Test

A Pap smear is a procedure the removes samples of cells from the cervix to assess if there are any abnormal cells. The sample is sent to the laboratory for microscopic identification. Further examination is necessary if the sample is positive, indicating abnormal cells on the cervix.

A negative Pap smear result does not mean that the patient is free from cervical cancer. It means that no abnormal cells were contained in the tissue sample. Abnormal cells might exist in areas of the cervix that was not sampled.

16.4 Vaginosis Tests

Vaginosis tests are used to assess the cause of vaginal itching, inflammation, and discharge, and identify the treatment for vaginosis.

Understanding the Vaginosis Tests

Vaginosis is the inflammation of the vulva and vagina caused by an infection or a reaction to an irritant, resulting in painful vaginal discharge and itching. The most common causes of vaginosis are:

- ***Candida albicans*:** This is a yeast infection that causes lumpy white discharge and itching.
- ***Trichomonas vaginalis*:** This causes a foamy yellow-green odorous vaginal discharge.
- ***Bacterial vaginosis*:** This causes a milky thick vaginal discharge that gives off a fishy odor.

Vaginosis tests are performed by the health care provider to sample the vaginal discharge and send the sample to a laboratory for examination. There are four vaginosis tests:

1. **Whiff Test:** Potassium hydroxide solution is dropped on the sample. If a fishy odor emanates, then the patient has bacterial vaginosis.
2. **KOH Slide:** The sample is mixed with potassium hydroxide solution. Only the yeast remains on the slide, indicating that the patient has a yeast infection.
3. **Wet Mount:** The sample is mixed with saline on a slide. The laboratory technician then identifies through microscopic examination the organism that is causing the infection.
4. **Vaginal pH:** The pH level of the sample is tested. A pH level >4.5 indicates bacterial vaginosis.

16.5 Sperm Penetration Tests

The sperm penetration tests are used to assess the underlying cause of infertility.

Understanding the Sperm Penetration Tests

Sperm penetration tests are performed when a woman is having difficulty becoming pregnant to determine if the sperm can move through the cervical mucus and into the fallopian tubes. There are two types of sperm penetration tests:

1. **Sperm Penetration Assay:** This test mixes sperm with hamster eggs to see if the sperm can penetrate the egg. The result is measured as a sperm capacitation index.
2. **Sperm Mucus Penetration:** This test determines if sperm can move through the cervical mucus.

Solved Problems

Female Tests

16.1 What is the purpose of the BRCA test?

The BRCA test is used to assess the patient's chances of developing breast or ovarian cancer.

16.2 What is BRCA?

Two genes called the breast cancer genes are BRCA1 and BRCA2, and they are associated with breast and ovarian cancer.

16.3 How would you respond to a patient who has the BRCA genes and who said that she is going to develop breast cancer?

A patient who carries this mutated gene and who has a family history of breast or ovarian cancer may have a higher than normal chance of developing breast cancer or ovarian cancer. However, the patient also has a chance of not developing these cancers.

16.4 What does the BRCA test assess?

The breast cancer gene test determines if the patient's BRCA1 and BRCA2 genes are mutated.

16.5 What might the health care provider suggest if the patient tests positive for BRCA?

The patient who tests positive may be advised to take tamoxifen to inhibit this gene.

16.6 How would you respond if a male patient says it is impossible for him to have the BRCA gene?

Male patients who have a family history of breast and prostate cancer may also have this gene. These patients can also develop breast and prostate cancer.

16.7 What is the purpose of the Pap smear?

The Pap smear is used to assess cervical tissue and identify abnormal cervical tissues that might be cancerous.

16.8 How is a Pap smear performed?

A Pap smear is a procedure that removes sample cells from the cervix to assess if there are any abnormal cells. The sample is sent to the laboratory for microscopic identification.

16.9 What is meant by a negative Pap smear?

It means that no abnormal cells were contained in the tissue sample.

16.10 Can a patient have a negative Pap smear and still have cervical cancer?

Yes, because cancerous cells might not have been sampled.

16.11 What is the purpose of the vaginosis test?

The vaginosis tests are used to assess the cause of vaginal itchy inflammation and discharge, and identify the treatment for vaginosis.

16.12 What is vaginosis?

Vaginosis is the inflammation of the vulva and vagina caused by an infection or reaction to an irritant, resulting in a painful vaginal discharge and itching.

16.13 What is *Candida albicans*?

This is a yeast infection that causes lumpy white discharge and itching.

16.14 What is *Trichomonas vaginalis*?

This causes a foamy yellow-green odorous vaginal discharge.

16.15 What is bacterial vaginosis?

This causes a milky thick vaginal discharge that gives off a fishy odor.

16.16 What is the Whiff test?

This is a test in which potassium hydroxide solution is dropped on the sample. If a fishy odor emanates, then the patient has bacterial vaginosis.

16.17 What is the KOH slide test?

The KOH slide test is a test in which the sample is mixed with potassium hydroxide solution. Only the yeast remains on the slide, indicating that the patient has a yeast infection.

16.18 What is the wet mount test?

The wet mount test is a test in which the sample is mixed with saline on a slide. The laboratory technician then identifies through microscopic examination the organism causing the infection.

16.19 Why is the vaginal pH test?

The vaginal pH test is a test in which the pH level of the sample is tested. A pH level >4.5 indicates bacterial vaginosis.

16.20 What is the purpose of the sperm penetration tests?

The sperm penetration tests are used to assess the underlying cause of infertility.

16.21 When might the sperm penetration test be ordered?

Sperm penetration tests are performed when a woman is having difficulty becoming pregnant to determine if the sperm can move through the cervical mucus and into the fallopian tubes.

16.22 What is the sperm penetration assay test?

This test mixes sperm with hamster eggs to see if the sperm can penetrate the egg.

16.23 What is the sperm mucus penetration test?

This test determines if sperm can move through the cervical mucus.

16.24 How is the result of the sperm penetration assay test measured?

The result is measured as a sperm capacitation index.

16.25 Does a positive Pap smear test mean that the patient has cervical cancer?

No. The health care provider is likely to order further examinations and testing.

Maternity Tests

17.1 Definition

There are several tests that are performed during pregnancy and shortly after childbirth to assess the health of the fetus and newborn. In a high-risk pregnancy, the health care provider might perform a chorionic villus sampling or amniocentesis early on in the pregnancy to determine if the fetus has a genetic disorder or other health issues.

Amniocentesis, for example, may be suggested in high-risk pregnancies that have a high risk of birth defects. This condition is confirmed by performing a cordocentesis, in which a sample of blood is taken from the umbilical cord while in the womb.

Later in the pregnancy, the health care provider performs a biophysical profile of the fetus to determine the overall health of the fetus. This is where an assessment is made of the fetal heart rate, breathing and body movements, muscle tone, and the volume of amniotic fluid.

It is also around this same period when the mother may undergo a contraction stress test. The contraction stress test determines if the fetus is healthy enough to survive the reduced oxygen levels that are common with natural childbirth.

In some pregnancies, the woman might experience an incompetent cervix that could result in the cervix opening prior to the thirty-seventh week of gestation, causing a premature birth. In this situation, the health care provider is likely to perform a cervical cerclage, which temporarily closes the cervix until the mother enters labor.

If the birth is premature, the health care provider may perform a cranial ultrasound to determine if there were complications caused by the premature birth. The newborn is typically administered the sweat test that helps determine if the newborn has a high level of chloride in his or her sweat, which may be an indication of cystic fibrosis.

17.2 Biophysical Profile (BPP) Test

This test is performed to assess:

- Fetal movement
- Fetal heart rate
- Volume of amniotic fluid
- Muscle tone
- Fetal breathing rate

Understanding the Biophysical Profile Test

The biophysical profile (BPP) test assesses the health of the fetus and is commonly performed in the last trimester of the pregnancy, although the health care provider may perform this test earlier and more frequently in high-risk pregnancies. The biophysical profile test consists of a nonstress test and a fetal ultrasound. Each element of the test is graded according to the following table:

Biophysical Profile Test

	NONSTRESS TEST	BREATHING MOVEMENT	BODY MOVEMENT	MUSCLE TONE	AMNIOTIC FLUID VOLUME
Normal (2 points)	2 or more heart rate increases with a rate of 15 minutes or greater while the fetus moves	1 or more breathing movements of 60 seconds	3 or more arm, leg, or body movement	Flexed arms and legs. Head rests on chest. 1 or more extensions and flexion	1 cm of amniotic fluid in the uterine cavity
Abnormal (0 points)	1 or more heart rate increases or the rate is not 15 minutes or greater while the fetus moves	Breathing movements of less than 60 seconds	Less than 3 arm, leg, or body movements	Arms, legs, and spine are extended. Open hand. Fetus not returning to normal position. Extension and flexion are slow	Less than 1 cm of amniotic fluid in the uterine cavity

17.3 Contraction Stress Test

The contraction stress test assesses the health of the placenta and the ability of the fetus to remain healthy during natural childbirth.

Understanding the Contraction Stress Test

The health care provider usually performs a biophysical profile of the fetus to assess breathing, movement, muscle tone, and the volume of amniotic fluid. If the biophysical profile indicates suspicious results, then the health care provider might perform a contraction stress test.

The contraction stress test determines if the fetus will remain healthy during natural childbirth. Uterine contractions reduce oxygen to the fetus, which normally does not harm the fetus. However, some fetuses can become negatively affected by the lower oxygen level so the health care provider might decide on a cesarean birth.

During the contraction stress test a fetal heart monitor is attached to the mother while the mother is administered oxytocin. Oxytocin is a hormone that induces uterine contractions. The fetal heart rate is expected to decelerate during a contraction and accelerate following the contraction. If the heart rate does not accelerate, then the fetus may not remain healthy during natural childbirth.

This test is not usually performed if the mother had a cesarean section in the past, placenta previa, placenta abruptio, incompetent cervix, premature rupture of the amniotic membrane, administered magnesium sulfate, or is pregnant with multiple fetuses.

17.4 Cranial Ultrasound Test

The cranial ultrasound test assesses the underlying cause of an enlarged head and assesses for:

- Hydrocephalus
- Risk of developing cerebral palsy
- Intraventricular hemorrhage
- Periventricular leukomalacia

Understanding the Cranial Ultrasound Test

A cranial ultrasound is performed on premature newborns to assess complications that might have arisen during the premature birth. During a cranial ultrasound, images of the newborn's brain are captured, displayed on a computer screen, and stored in a computer. The health care provider might order several cranial ultrasounds weeks apart. Some complications such as intraventricular hemorrhage (IVH) can be detected during the first week of birth, while other complications such as periventricular leukomalacia (PVL) might occur 8 weeks after birth. Periventricular leukomalacia is damaged tissue around the ventricles.

A cranial ultrasound is not performed after the child is 18 months of age because the cranium is fully formed and the fontanelle is closed.

17.5 Amniocentesis

Amniocentesis is ordered to assess fetal lung development and assess:

- Birth defects
- Chorioamnionitis
- Rh antibodies

Understanding the Amniocentesis Test

Amniotic fluid contains cells shed by the fetus. At about the sixteenth week of gestation, the health care provider may perform amniocentesis, which is the removal of some amniotic fluid. Fetal cells contain amniotic fluid and are analyzed to determine if the fetus has a birth defect. Amniocentesis is also performed during the third trimester if there is a risk of premature birth to determine fetal lung development and assess if the mother has chorioamnionitis, which is infection of the amniotic fluid.

Amniocentesis is ordered if an integrated test is positive, indicating that the fetus has a high chance of having a birth defect. This test includes alpha-fetoprotein (AFP), estriol, inhibin A, and human chorionic gonadotropin (hCG). It is also ordered if parents are carriers of a genetic trait that is likely to be passed on to the fetus. These include cystic fibrosis, Duchenne muscular dystrophy, sickle cell anemia, thalassemia, hemophilia, and Tay-Sachs disease.

Amniocentesis is also performed to determine if the fetus is Rh positive when the mother has the Rh factor. This tests the amniotic fluid for increased bilirubin levels after the twentieth week of gestation, which indicates that the fetal blood cells are being attacked by the mother's antibodies.

Amniocentesis does not identify all birth defects. There are many birth defects that are not revealed by amniocentesis.

17.6 Cordocentesis Test

The cordocentesis test assesses the oxygen level in fetal blood, assesses for fetal anemia, and if the fetus is Rh positive.

Understanding the Cordocentesis Test

If amniocentesis or other tests reveal that the fetus might have anemia, the health provider may order a cordocentesis to confirm the finding, typically in the second trimester. A cordocentesis is the sampling of fetal blood from the umbilical cord to determine if the fetus has a blood disorder or is Rh positive. The blood sample is also used to assess the oxygen level in fetal blood.

17.7 Sweat Test

The sweat test assesses for cystic fibrosis.

Understanding the Sweat Test

The sweat test is administered to a newborn between the age of 2 days and 5 months old to assess if the newborn might have cystic fibrosis. Children who have cystic fibrosis have increased sodium chloride in their sweat. The sweat test measures the amount of chloride in sweat.

17.8 Chorionic Villus Sampling (CVS) Test

The chorionic villus sampling (CVS) test assesses for fetal genetic disorders.

Understanding the Chorionic Villus Sampling Test

The placenta contains chorionic villi, which are tiny growths that contain the same genetic material as the fetus. CVS is a procedure where a sampling of chorionic villi is biopsied between the tenth and twelfth weeks of gestation and examined to determine if the fetus has a genetic disorder. There are two methods used to biopsy the chorionic villus:

1. **Transabdominal:** A needle is inserted through the abdomen.
2. **Transcervical:** A needle is inserted through the cervix.

Chorionic villus sampling is performed earlier in gestation than amniocentesis.

17.9 Karyotyping

The karyotyping test assesses for fetal genetic disorders.

Understanding the Karyotyping Test

Karyotyping is a test that determines the number and quality of chromosomes in a cell and is used to detect possible genetic disorders. Tissue samples for karyotyping are typically taken during CVS or amniocentesis.

17.10 Cervical Cerclage (Weak Cervix)

The cervical cerclage prevents premature opening of the cervix.

Understanding the Cervical Cerclage

If the patient has an incompetent cervix, the cervix might open prior to the thirty-seventh week of gestation and could result in premature birth. The health care provider may perform a cervical cerclage, which is a procedure to close the cervix, to assure that the cervix remains closed until after the thirty-seventh week of gestation.

The cervix must be manually opened before the patient goes into labor; otherwise, the health care provider may perform a cesarean section.

17.11 Galactosemia Test

The galactosemia test is ordered to screen for galactosemia.

Understanding the Galactosemia Test

A newborn who has galactosemia may experience seizures, brain damage, and mental retardation if its body is unable to convert galactose, which is found in breast milk and formula, into glucose. This is because the newborn lacks three enzymes needed for this process. The galactosemia test determines if these enzymes are present in the newborn's blood.

These enzymes can also be detected in a urine sample.

Solved Problems

Maternity Tests

17.1 Why would the health care provider order the biophysical profile (BPP) test?

The biophysical profile (BPP) test is performed to assess fetal movement, fetal heart rate, volume of amniotic fluid, muscle tone, and fetal breathing rate.

17.2 When is the BPP test performed?

The BPP test is commonly performed in the last trimester of pregnancy, although the health care provider may perform this test earlier and more frequently in high-risk pregnancies.

17.3 Of what does the BPP test consist?

The BPP test consists of a nonstress test and a fetal ultrasound.

17.4 What does the BPP test measure?

The BPP test measures breathing movements, body movements, muscle tone, and amniotic fluid volume.

17.5 What is considered abnormal body movement in the BPP test?

Abnormal body movement in the BPP test is <3 arm, leg, or body movements.

17.6 What is the purpose of the contraction stress test?

The contraction stress test assesses the health of the placenta and the ability of the fetus to remain healthy during natural childbirth.

17.7 When might the contraction stress test be ordered?

The contraction stress test might be performed if the result of the BPP is abnormal.

17.8 Why might a fetus be adversely affected by natural childbirth?

Uterine contractions reduce oxygen to the fetus, which normally does not harm the fetus. However, some fetuses can become negatively affected by the lower oxygen level.

17.9 How is the contraction stress test performed?

During the contraction stress test, a fetal heart monitor is attached to the mother while the mother is administered oxytocin. Oxytocin is a hormone that induces uterine contractions. The fetal heart rate is expected to decelerate during a contraction and accelerate following the contraction. If the heart rate does not accelerate, the fetus may not remain healthy during natural childbirth.

17.10 When is the contraction stress test not performed?

This test is not usually performed if the mother in the past has had a caesarean section, placenta previa, placenta abruptio, incompetent cervix, premature rupture of the amniotic membrane, administered magnesium sulfate, or is pregnant with multiple fetuses.

17.11 When might amniocentesis be performed?

At about the sixteenth week of gestation, the health care provider may perform amniocentesis. Amniocentesis is also performed during the third trimester if there is a risk of premature birth to determine fetal lung development and assess if the mother has chorioamnionitis.

17.12 Why might the health care provider order an amniocentesis?

Amniotic fluid contains cells shed by the fetus. Fetal cells contain amniotic fluid and are analyzed to determine if the fetus has a birth defect. It is also ordered to assess if the mother has chorioamnionitis, which is infection of the amniotic fluid.

17.13 How does the health care provider know if fetal blood cells are being attacked by the mother's antibodies?

Amniocentesis is performed and the amniotic fluid is examined for increased bilirubin levels after the twentieth week of gestation, which indicates that the fetal blood cells are being attacked by the mother's antibodies.

17.14 When might amniocentesis be ordered?

Amniocentesis is ordered if an integrated test is positive, indicating that the fetus has a high chance of having a birth defect. This test includes alpha-fetoprotein (AFP), estriol, inhibin A, and human chorionic gonadotropin (hCG). It is also ordered if parents are carriers of a genetic trait that is likely to be passed on to the fetus. These include cystic fibrosis, Duchenne muscular dystrophy, sickle cell anemia, thalassemia, hemophilia, and Tay-Sachs disease.

17.15 If the amniocentesis is negative, does it mean that the fetus is free from birth defects?

No. Amniocentesis does not identify all birth defects. There are many birth defects that are not revealed by amniocentesis.

17.16 What is the purpose of the cordocentesis test?

The cordocentesis test assesses the oxygen level in fetal blood, assesses for fetal anemia, and assesses if the fetus is Rh positive.

17.17 How is the cordocentesis test performed?

A cordocentesis is the sampling of fetal blood from the umbilical cord to determine if the fetus has a blood disorder or is Rh positive. The blood sample is also used to assess the oxygen level in fetal blood.

17.18 What is the purpose of the sweat test?

The sweat test assesses for cystic fibrosis.

17.19 How is the sweat test performed?

The sweat test measures the amount of chloride in sweat.

17.20 When is the sweat test administered?

The sweat test is administered to a newborn between 2 days and 5 months old.

17.21 When is the chorionic villus sampling (CVS) test performed?

CVS is performed between the tenth and twelfth weeks of gestation.

17.22 What are chorionic villi?

The placenta contains chorionic villi, which are tiny growths that contain the same genetic material as the fetus.

17.23 What is the advantage of the CVS test over amniocentesis?

The CVS test can be performed earlier in gestation than amniocentesis.

17.24 What is a transabdominal CVS test?

A transabdominal CVS test occurs when the sampling of the placenta is taken by inserting a needle through the abdomen.

17.25 What is a transcervical CVS test?

A transcervical CVS test occurs when the sampling of the placenta is taken by inserting a needle through the cervix.

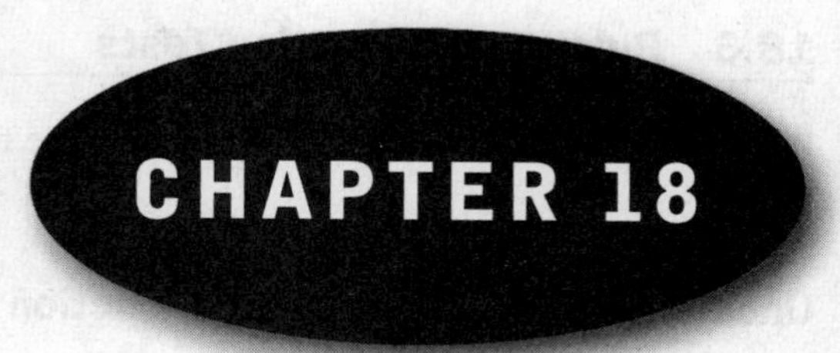

CHAPTER 18

Chest, Abdominal, and Urinary Tract Tests

18.1 Definition

When there are suspected disorders of the upper gastrointestinal tract, thyroid gland, liver, gallbladder, kidney, spleen, urinary tract, and other organs in the upper part of the body, the health care provider is likely to order a number of tests to uncover the underlying problem.

Some tests enable the health care provider to examine the esophagus, stomach, duodenum, bile, and pancreatic ducts and to take a biopsy, or, in some cases, remove an obstruction. Other tests enable the health care provider to scan the liver, spleen, gallbladder, and kidney by using contrast material to highlight the structure of the organ. Images of the organ are captured with a camera and studied to uncover diseases and disorders.

There are also procedures that the health care provider can perform to temporarily or permanently repair a problem. Some examples are the removal of a cancerous thyroid gland, a tumor from the bladder, or fixing urinary incontinence.

18.2 Lung Scan

The lung scan is used to assess blood flow to the lungs and identify a pulmonary embolism.

Understanding the Lung Scan

A lung scan is performed to detect a pulmonary embolism that impedes blood flow to the lungs. There are three types of lung scans:

1. **Perfusion:** In a perfusion scan, the patient is injected with a radioactive tracer into a blood vessel. An image is taken of the lungs as the tracer circulates to the lungs. A pulmonary embolism is suspected in areas of the lung where the tracer is not seen.
2. **Ventilation:** In a ventilation scan, the patient inhales gas that contains a radioactive tracer. An image is taken of the lungs. A pulmonary embolism is suspected in areas of the lung that are not receiving the tracer.
3. **V/Q:** A V/Q scan consists of both the perfusion and the ventilation scan. The ventilation scan is performed first. This is the most commonly performed lung scan.

18.3 Pulmonary Function Tests

Pulmonary function tests are used to assess the function of the patient's lungs and monitor progress of lung therapy.

Understanding the Pulmonary Function Tests

There are a number of pulmonary function tests used to assess how well the patient's lungs perform. These tests are:

- **Gas Diffusion:** Measures the amount of gasses that cross the alveoli per minute. These include arterial blood gases and the carbon monoxide diffusing capacity.
- **Spirometry:** This measures the volume and capacity of the lungs. The patient breathes into a mouthpiece of the spirometer, and information measured by the spirometer is printed out in a chart called a spirogram. Common lung function values that are measured are:
  - *Forced vital capacity (FVC):* Amount of forced exhaled air
  - *Forced expiratory volume (FEV):* Amount of exhaled air with force in one breath measured in seconds
  - *Forced expiratory flow 25 to 75%:* Air flow halfway through an exhale
  - *Peak expiratory flow (PEF):* Air quickly exhaled
  - *Maximum voluntary ventilation (MVV):* Greatest amount of air the patient breathes in and out in 1 minute
  - *Slow vital capacity (SVC):* Amount of air slowly exhaled after inhaling as deeply as possible
  - *Total lung capacity (TLC):* Amount of air in lungs after inhaling as deeply as possible
  - *Functional residual capacity (FRC):* Amount of air in lungs at the end of a normal exhaled breath
  - *Residual volume (RV):* Amount of air in lungs after exhaled completely
  - *Expiratory reserve volume (ERV):* The difference between the amount of air in the lungs after a normal exhale (FRC) and the amount after exhaled with force (FVC)
- **Exercise Stress:** Measures the effect exercise has on the lungs
- **Body Plethysmograph:** Measures the volume and capacity of the lungs
- **Inhalation Challenge:** Assesses the patient's airway responses to allergens

18.4 Upper Gastrointestinal (UGI) Test Series

The upper gastrointestinal (UGI) test is used to assess the underlying cause of stomach pain and indigestion and the underlying cause of malabsorption syndrome.

Understanding the Upper Gastrointestinal Test Series

The upper gastrointestinal test series consists of a group of tests that assess the esophagus, stomach, and duodenum. Prior to the series, the patient ingests barium contrast material and water. X-ray images of the esophagus, stomach, and duodenum are taken using a fluoroscope as the barium moves through the UGI tract. Images are displayed on a computer screen and stored for further review. If the health care provider sees anything suspicious, he or she might perform an endoscopy, in which an endoscope is inserted down the esophagus and into the stomach and duodenum to directly view the UGI tract.

The UGI series is also performed during a full gastrointestinal series, which also involves examination of the lower gastrointestinal tract.

18.5 Esophagus Test Series

The esophagus test series is used to assess the underlying cause of gastroesophageal reflux (GER) and chest pain.

Understanding the Esophagus Test Series

The esophagus test series consists of two tests that assess the esophagus and esophageal sphincters:

1. **Esophageal Manometry:** Measures esophageal muscle contractions
2. **Esophageal Acidity Test:** Measures the pH of the esophagus

18.6 Gallbladder Scan

The gallbladder scan is used to assess the structure of the gallbladder and the underlying cause of upper right abdominal pain.

Understanding the Gallbladder Scan

A gallbladder scan assesses the function of the gallbladder and is used to identify blockages in the bile ducts. A radioactive tracer is injected into the patient's vein. The tracer is removed from the blood by the liver, which places the tracer into bile that flows into the gallbladder and then the duodenum. A camera takes an image of the tracer as the tracer flows through the liver to the duodenum.

18.7 Kidney Scan

The kidney scan is used to assess blood flow through the kidneys and kidney function.

Understanding the Kidney Scan

A kidney scan assesses the function of the kidney. A radioactive tracer is injected into the patient's vein. The tracer moves through the blood vessels into the kidneys. A camera takes an image of the tracer as the tracer flows through the kidney, illustrating where blood flows unobstructed and where blood flow is blocked. There are two types of kidney scans:

1. **Function Study:** This measures the time that the tracer takes to pass through the kidneys and enter the bladder as part of urine.
2. **Perfusion Study:** This assesses blood flow through the kidneys.

A kidney scan is an alternative to the intravenous pyelogram (IVP) test.

18.8 Liver and Spleen Scan

The liver and spleen scan assesses blood flow through the liver and spleen. This scan also assesses the spleen following an injury and the liver to determine if cancer has metastasized to the liver. The liver and spleen scan is also used to assess cancer treatment.

Understanding the Liver and Spleen Scan

A liver and spleen scan assesses the function of the liver and spleen. A radioactive tracer is injected into the patient's vein. The tracer moves through the blood vessels in the liver and spleen. A camera takes an image of the tracer as the tracer flows through the liver and spleen, illustrating where blood flows unobstructed and where blood flow is blocked.

18.9 Urinalysis

Urinalysis is performed to assess kidney function and other disorders.

Understanding Urinalysis

Waste material carried by blood is filtered by kidneys and excreted as urine. A urinalysis is performed to determine the characteristics of the urine and the existence and amount of substances in the urine. Urine characteristics are:

- **Clarity:** How clear is the urine?
- **Color:** What color is the urine?
- **Specific Gravity:** The balance between water and substances in the urine
- **Odor:** The aroma of urine
- **pH:** How acidic or alkaline is the urine?

There are several methods used to capture the urine sample:

- **Clean-Catch Midstream One-Time Urine Collection:** Urine is collected after the patient begins to urinate.
- **Double-Voided Urine Collection:** Urine is collected the second time that the patient voids.
- **24-Hour Urine Collection:** Urine is collected over a 24-hour period.

18.10 Urine Culture and Sensitivity Test

The urine culture and sensitivity test is performed to assess the existence and type of microorganism in a patient with a urinary tract infection (UTI), as well as the proper medication to prescribe treatment.

Understanding the Urine Culture and Sensitivity Test

A urine culture is ordered when the patient is suspected of having a UTI. A urine collection is placed in an environment conducive to the growth of microorganisms for 3 days. The urine is examined to identify the presence and type of microorganism. Once the microorganism is identified, a sensitivity test is performed to determine the medication that kills the microorganism.

18.11 Renin Assay Test

The renin assay test is ordered to determine the underlying cause of hypertension.

Understanding the Renin Assay Test

The renin assay test is performed with the aldosterone test to determine the underlying cause of hypertension. Renin is an enzyme produced by the kidneys. Aldosterone is a hormone produced by the adrenal glands. Together, these work to balance the sodium and potassium levels within the patient. A high renin level might indicate a kidney disorder. A low renin level might indicate Conn's syndrome. A low renin level and a high aldosterone level might indicate an adrenal gland tumor.

18.12 Thyroid Scan

The thyroid scan is used to assess thyroid function and the treatment for thyroid disease.

Understanding the Thyroid Scan Test

A thyroid scan assesses the function of the thyroid gland. There are two types of thyroid scans:

1. **Radioactive Iodine Uptake (RAIU) Test:** This assesses the absorption of a radioactive tracer by the thyroid gland.
2. **Whole-Body Thyroid Scan:** This test assesses whether or not thyroid cancer metastasized.

18.13 Thyroid and Parathyroid Ultrasound

The thyroid and parathyroid ultrasound assesses the size and shape of the thyroid and parathyroid glands.

Understanding the Thyroid and Parathyroid Ultrasound

The thyroid and parathyroid ultrasound is used to assess the size and shape of the thyroid gland and the parathyroid glands, which are located behind the thyroid gland. This test is not used to assess the function of these glands.

18.14 Thyroid Hormone Tests

The thyroid hormone tests are used to assess for hyper- and hypothyroidism, and the underlying cause of abnormal thyroid-stimulating hormone (TSH) test results. It is also used to assess treatment of hyper- and hypothyroidism.

Understanding the Thyroid Hormone Tests

The thyroid produces two hormones: thyroxine (T4) and triiodothyronine (T3). The thyroid hormone tests measure the levels of thyroid hormones in the patient's blood. There are three thyroid hormone tests:

1. **Free Thyroxine (FT4):** This test determines the amount of thyroxine that is not bound to globulin.
2. **Total Thyroxine (T4):** This test determines the total amount of thyroxine that is attached to globulin and not bound to globulin.
3. **Triiodothyronine (T3):** This test determines the total amount of triiodothyronine that is attached to globulin and not bound to globulin.

18.15 Thyroid-Stimulating Hormone (TSH) Test

The thyroid-stimulating hormone (TSH) test is ordered to assess the underlying cause of hyper- and hypothyroidism.

Understanding the Thyroid-Stimulating Hormone Test

The hypothalamus produces thyrotropin-releasing hormone (TRH), which causes the pituitary gland to produce the TSH. This causes the thyroid to produce thyroid hormones.

18.16 Salivary Gland Scan

The salivary gland scan assesses the function of the salivary glands and the underlying cause of swollen salivary glands and dry mouth.

Understanding the Salivary Gland Scan

A small amount of radioactive tracer is injected into the patient's vein. Every few minutes an image is taken with a camera that detects the tracer in the bloodstream of the salivary gland. The patient is requested to suck on a lemon to cause the salivary glands to release saliva and increase the image of the salivary gland. Any blockage appears on the image.

18.17 D-Xylose Absorption Test

The D-xylose absorption test assesses the intestine's ability to absorb D-xylose.

Understanding the D-Xylose Absorption Test

Patients with malabsorption syndrome are unable to absorb certain nutrients into their blood from the intestinal tract. This can result in malnutrition and chronic diarrhea. The D-xylose absorption test assesses whether or not these signs are a result of malabsorption syndrome by asking the patient to drink a solution of D-xylose and then measuring the amount of D-xylose in the patient's blood and urine.

18.18 Stool Culture

A stool culture is ordered to identify microorganism in a stool sample.

Understanding the Stool Culture

A patient may exhibit diarrhea and other signs of an infection. The health care provider orders a stool culture to determine if the underlying cause is a microorganism. A sample of the patient's stool is sent to the laboratory where it is placed in an environment that encourages the microorganism to grow. After 3 days, laboratory technicians determine if a microorganism is present and, if so, which microorganism.

The health care provider typically orders a sensitivity test of the sample along with the stool culture. The sensitivity test determines the medication that kills the microorganism.

18.19 Entero-Test (Giardiasis String Test)

The Entero-Test is used to detect the presence of *Giardia intestinalis.*

Understanding the Entero-Test

A patient who has severe diarrhea might have giardiasis. Giardiasis is caused by an intestinal parasite called *Giardia intestinalis* that is found in water, food, or soil that is contaminated with feces. The Entero-Test determines if the patient has giardiasis by sampling fluid in the duodenum. The patient swallows a gelatin capsule that is attached to a string. The string is taped to the outside of the patient's mouth while the capsule dissolves in the stomach and the duodenum. The string is then removed and examined under a microscope.

18.20 Stool Analysis

The stool analysis is used to assess:

- Digestive tract disorder
- Liver disorder
- Pancreas disorder
- Colon cancer
- Absorption disorder

Understanding Stool Analysis

A stool analysis is the examination of the patient's feces to identify digestive tract disorders. The patient's stool sample is examined for color, volume, consistency, odor, and the presence of blood, fat, mucus, fiber, bile, and glucose.

18.21 Fecal Occult Blood Test (FOBT)

The fecal occult blood test (FOBT) is used to identify blood in the stool.

Understanding the Fecal Occult Blood Test

Blood in stool is not always visible. The FOBT examines the stool for blood that is not visible to the naked eye. This is referred to as occult blood. Although the presence of occult blood is linked to colon cancer, there are many other causes of occult blood in stool.

18.22 Overnight Dexamethasone Suppression Test

The overnight dexamethasone suppression test is used to screen for Cushing's syndrome.

Understanding the Overnight Dexamethasone Suppression Test

The pituitary glands secrete adrenocorticotropic hormone (ACTH) based on the amount of cortisol in the patient's blood. ACTH signals the adrenal glands to secrete cortisol. In Cushing's syndrome, cortisol is secreted regardless of the secretion of the ACTH level. The overnight dexamethasone suppression test requires the patient to take dexamethasone, which is a corticosteroid. This increases the cortisol level in the patient's blood and therefore signals the pituitary glands not to secrete ACTH and, as a result, the adrenal glands should not secrete cortisol. In the morning, the patient's cortisol level should be relatively low. If not, then the patient might have Cushing's syndrome.

Solved Problems

Chest, Abdominal, and Urinary Tract Tests

18.1 What is the purpose of a lung scan?

The lung scan is used to assess blood flow to the lungs and identify a pulmonary embolism.

18.2 What is a perfusion scan?

In a perfusion scan, the patient is injected with a radioactive tracer into a blood vessel. An image is taken of the lungs as the tracer circulates to the lungs. A pulmonary embolism is suspected in areas of the lung where the tracer is not seen.

18.3 What is a ventilation scan?

In a ventilation scan, the patient inhales gas that contains a radioactive tracer. An image is taken of the lungs. A pulmonary embolism is suspected in areas of the lung that are not receiving the tracer.

18.4 What is a V/Q scan?

A V/Q scan consists of both the perfusion scan and the ventilation scan. The ventilation scan is performed first. This is the most commonly performed lung scan.

18.5 What are gas diffusion tests?

Gas diffusion tests measure the amount of gases that cross the alveoli per minute. These include arterial blood gases and the carbon monoxide diffusing capacity.

18.6 What is the body plethysmograph test?

The body plethysmograph test measures the volume and capacity of the lungs.

18.7 Why is an upper gastrointestinal (UGI) series ordered?

The upper gastrointestinal (UGI) test series is used to assess the underlying cause of stomach pain and indigestion and the underlying cause of malabsorption syndrome.

18.8 How is a UGI series performed?

The UGI series consists of a group of tests that assess the esophagus, stomach, and duodenum. Prior to the series, the patient ingests barium contrast material and water. X-ray images of the esophagus, stomach, and duodenum are taken using a fluoroscope as the barium moves through the UGI tract. Images are displayed on a computer screen and stored for further review. If the health care provider sees anything suspicious, he or she might perform an endoscopy, in which an endoscope is inserted down the esophagus and into the stomach and duodenum to directly view the UGI tract.

18.9 What is the purpose of the esophagus test series?

The esophagus test series is used to assess the underlying cause of gastroesophageal reflux (GER) and chest pain.

18.10 What is the purpose of the esophageal manometry?

Esophageal manometry measures esophageal muscle contractions.

18.11 How is a gallbladder scan performed?

A gallbladder scan assesses the function of the gallbladder and is used to identify blockages in the bile ducts. A radioactive tracer is injected into the patient's vein. The tracer is removed from the blood by the liver, which places the tracer into bile that flows into the gallbladder and duodenum. A camera takes an image of the tracer as the tracer flows through the liver to the duodenum.

18.12 What is the purpose of a urinalysis?

Waste material carried by blood is filtered by kidneys and excreted as urine. A urinalysis is performed to determine the characteristics of the urine and the existence and amount of substances in the urine.

18.13 What are the characteristics of urine?

- **Clarity:** How clear is the urine?
- **Color:** What is the color of the urine?
- **Specific Gravity:** The balance between water and substances in the urine
- **Odor:** The aroma of urine
- **pH:** How acidic or alkaline is the urine?

18.14 What is a double-voided urine collection?

The double-voided urine collection is urine collected the second time the patient voids.

18.15 What is a clean-catch midstream one-time urine collection?

The clean-catch midstream one-time urine collection is urine is collected after the patient begins to urinate.

18.16 What would you expect a health care provider to order if he or she suspects a urinary tract infection (UTI)?

The urine culture and sensitivity test is performed to assess the existence and type of microorganism in a patient with a UTI and is also used to assess the proper medication to prescribe to treat the UTI.

18.17 What is the purpose of the renin assay test?

The renin assay test is ordered to determine the underlying cause of hypertension.

18.18 How is the renin assay test performed?

The renin assay test is performed with the aldosterone test to determine the underlying cause of hypertension. Renin is an enzyme produced by the kidneys. Aldosterone is a hormone produced by the adrenal glands. Together, these work to balance the sodium and potassium levels in the patient.

18.19 What is the radioactive iodine uptake (RAIU) test?

The RAIU test assesses the absorption of a radioactive tracer by the thyroid gland.

18.20 Why might the whole-body thyroid scan be ordered?

This test assesses whether or not thyroid cancer metastasized.

18.21 Why are thyroid hormone tests ordered?

Thyroid hormone tests are used to assess for hyper- and hypothyroidism and for the underlying cause of abnormal thyroid-stimulating hormone (TSH) test results. They are also used to assess treatment of hyper- and hypothyroidism.

18.22 What is the free thyroxine test?

The free thyroxine (FT4) test determines the amount of thyroxine that is not bound to globulin.

18.23 What is the total thyroxine test?

The total thyroxine (T4) test determines the total amount of thyroxine that is attached to globulin and not bound to globulin.

18.24 What is the purpose of the thyroid-stimulating hormone (TSH) test?

The thyroid-stimulating hormone (TSH) test determines the underlying cause of thyroid disorder.

18.25 What is the purpose of the D-xylose absorption test?

The D-xylose absorption test assesses the intestine's ability to absorb D-xylose.

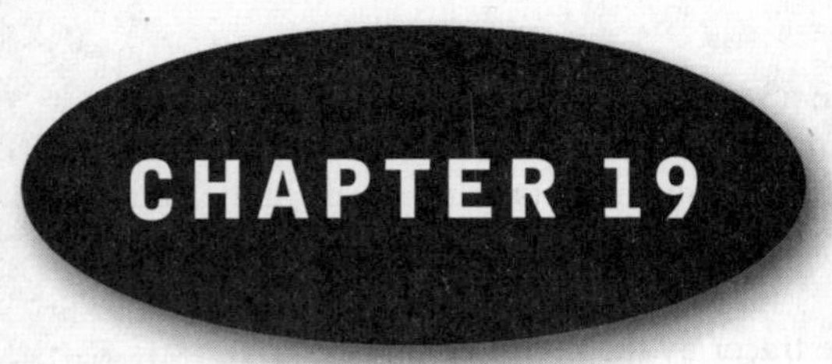

Male Tests

19.1 Definition

There are a number of medical tests and procedures that are specifically designed to diagnose and treat disorders that affect men. There are a group of tests and procedures focused on fertility.

When a man is unable to impregnate a woman, the health care provider orders tests to assess if there is an underlying problem with the man's reproductive organs. The initial test is a semen analysis that assesses the man's semen and sperm. Depending on the results, a testicular scan or ultrasound is ordered to determine if there is a structural disorder. One such structural disorder is varicocele, which is a large vein that blocks blood flow to the testicles. This is relieved by performing a varicocele repair.

The health care provider may follow up with a testicular examination or an erectile dysfunction test. If the erectile dysfunction test returns positive results, the health care provider may perform a penile implant procedure in which a device is inserted to cause an erection.

Some men desire to become infertile by having their vas deferens cut or blocked by a vasectomy. This prevents sperm from mixing with semen, resulting in no sperm in the ejaculate. A vasectomy in some instances can be reversed by performing a vasovasostomy.

Men are susceptible to developing an enlarged prostate gland, which could be caused by prostate cancer. Prostatic cancer cells are in part fueled by testosterone, which is produced by the testicles. The health care provider might perform an orchiectomy, which is the surgical removal of one or both testicles. This reduces the level of testosterone in the patient's body.

Alternatively, the health care provider may perform a prostatectomy, which is the removal of the prostate gland. However, this procedure may leave the patient with erectile dysfunction and urinary incontinence.

19.2 Erectile Dysfunction Tests

The erectile dysfunction test is performed to identify the underlying cause of erectile dysfunction.

Understanding Erectile Dysfunction Tests

Erectile dysfunction is commonly caused by psychological, blood vessel, and nerve disorders. There are three tests that are commonly ordered to assess erectile dysfunction:

1. **Color Duplex Doppler:** This test assesses blood flow through the penis using an ultrasound.
2. **Nocturnal Penile Tumescence (NPT):** This test assesses if the patient has erections during sleep.
3. **Intracavernosal Injection:** This test injects prostaglandin E1 into the base of the penis to cause an erection.

19.3 Testicular Ultrasound

The testicular ultrasound is ordered to identify the underlying cause of scrotum pain, and assess structures within the scrotum and a mass on the testicles.

Understanding the Testicular Ultrasound

A testicular ultrasound is a procedure used to produce an image of the testicles, scrotum, epididymis, and vas deferens to detect if there is any structural dysfunction.

19.4 Testicular Scan

A testicular scan assesses the function of the testicles and is used to identify blockages.

Understanding the Testicular Scan

A radioactive tracer is injected into the patient's vein. The tracer flows into the testicles. A camera takes an image of the tracer as the tracer flows through the testicles.

19.5 Semen Analysis

The semen analysis is ordered to identify the underlying cause of infertility and assess the results of a vasectomy and vasovasostomy. The health provider should inform the patient of the possibility of impregnating a woman for several weeks following a vasectomy. Only the semen analysis will determine when no sperm are mixing with the semen. It is at this time that the patient will be unable to impregnate a woman.

Understanding Semen Analysis

Semen analysis is performed to assess the volume of semen and number of quality sperm produced in an ejaculation to determine the underlying cause of infertility. Eight factors are analyzed:

1. **Semen Volume:** This is the amount of semen in an ejaculation.
2. **Liquefaction Time:** This is the time it takes for the semen to liquefy.
3. **Sperm Morphology:** This is the number of normally shaped sperm.
4. **Sperm Motility:** This is the percentage of sperm that show forward movement.
5. **Sperm Count:** This is the number of sperm in a milliliter of semen in one ejaculation.
6. **Fructose Level:** This is the amount of fructose in semen to provide energy for sperm.
7. **pH:** This measures the acidity level of the semen.
8. **Semen White Blood Cell Count:** This measures the number of white blood cells in semen, which is normally zero.

Solved Problems

Male Tests

19.1 What is a varicocele?

A varicocele is a large vein that blocks blood flow to the testicles.

19.2 What is a vasectomy?

A vasectomy is the cutting or blocking of the vas deferens to prevent sperm from mixing with semen.

19.3 What is the result of a successful vasectomy?

The result of a successful vasectomy is that no sperm are in the semen.

19.4 What is a vasovasostomy?

A vasovasostomy is a reversal of a vasectomy.

19.5 What are common causes of erectile dysfunction?

Erectile dysfunction is commonly caused by psychological, blood vessel, and nerve disorders.

19.6 What is a color duplex Doppler test?

This test assesses blood flow through the penis using an ultrasound.

19.7 What is the nocturnal penile tumescence test?

This test assesses if the patient has erections during sleep.

19.8 What is the intracavernosal injection test?

This test injects prostaglandin E1 into the base of the penis to cause an erection.

19.9 Why is a testicular ultrasound ordered?

The testicular ultrasound is ordered to identify the underlying cause of scrotum pain, and assess structures within the scrotum and a mass on the testicles.

19.10 What structures are viewed in a testicular ultrasound?

A testicular ultrasound is a procedure used to produce an image of the testicles, scrotum, epididymis, and vas deferens to detect if there is any structural dysfunction.

19.11 Why is a testicular scan ordered?

A testicular scan assesses the function of the testicles and is used to identify blockages.

19.12 How is a testicular scan performed?

A radioactive tracer is injected into the patient's vein. The tracer flows into the testicles. A camera takes an image of the tracer as the tracer flows through the testicles.

19.13 What test is ordered to assess the results of a vasectomy?

Semen analysis is ordered to assess the results of a vasectomy.

19.14 Why does a health care provider order semen analysis several weeks following a vasectomy?

It is common for sperm to mix with semen for several weeks following a vasectomy. The semen analysis determines when no sperm are in semen.

19.15 What will the health care provider tell the patient following a vasectomy regarding pregnancy?

The patient might be able to impregnate a woman for several weeks following a vasectomy. Only the semen analysis will determine when no sperm are mixing with the semen. It is at this time that the patient will be unable to impregnate a woman.

19.16 What other reason might a health care provider order a semen analysis?

The semen analysis is ordered to identify the underlying cause of infertility.

19.17 What does the semen volume test measure?

This is the amount of semen in an ejaculation.

19.18 What does the liquefaction time test measure?
This is the time it takes for the semen to liquefy.

19.19 What does the sperm morphology test measure?
This measures the number of normally shaped sperm.

19.20 What does the sperm motility test measure?
This is the percentage of sperm that show forward movement.

19.21 What does the sperm count test measure?
This is the number of sperm in a milliliter of semen in one ejaculation.

19.22 What does the fructose level measure?
This is the amount of fructose in semen to provide energy for sperm.

19.23 What does the pH test measure?
This measures the acidity level of the semen.

19.24 What does the semen white blood cell count measure?
This measures the number of white blood cells in semen.

19.25 What is the normal semen white blood cell count?
The normal semen white blood cell count is zero.

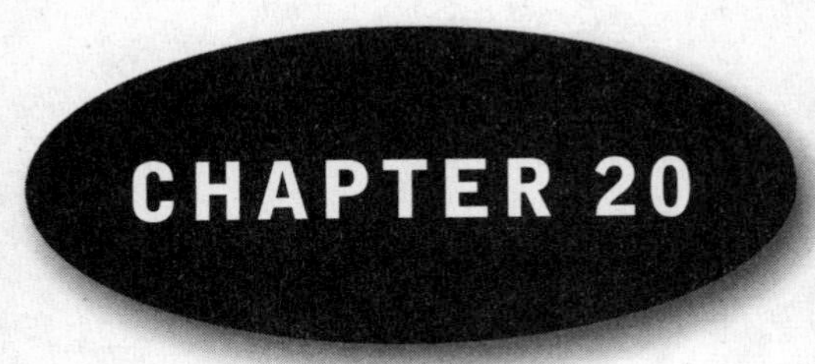

Skin Tests

20.1 Definition

Skin is the largest and most visible organ in the body and is susceptible to wrinkles, blemishes, growths (including both nonmelanoma and melanoma), and infection. Health care providers perform an assortment of tests and procedures to diagnose and treat skin conditions.

Lesions, warts, and blemishes that make skin unsightly and unhealthy can be removed by performing one of a number of procedures. For example, undesired tissue can be frozen with cryosurgery and removed, or layers of skin can be peeled away using chemicals or micrographic surgery. Layers can also be removed using curettage, electrosurgery, or the dermabrasion procedure in which a rotating burr scrapes scars and aging skin to encourage new skin growth.

Melanoma and nonmelanoma skin cancer affects many patients. The health care provider can cure or minimize the discomfort of this condition by performing a skin excision where the tumor is surgically removed.

Infected skin can be treated once the microorganism that causes the infection is identified. The health care provider is able to identify the microorganism by performing a wound culture in which a sample of the infected tissue is placed in an environment that is favorable for the growth of microorganism (culture) and then identified. Once the lab determines which medication will fight the microorganism, the medication is administered to the microorganism.

Skin is also a perfect site for testing for allergic reactions. There are several tests that health care providers administer to the skin to identify allergens that cause the patient to develop an allergic reaction. The skin is also the site of the Mantoux skin test to determine if the patient has ever been exposed to *Mycobacterium tuberculosis*.

20.2 Chemical Peel

A chemical peel is performed to cosmetically improve the patient's skin.

Understanding the Chemical Peel

A chemical peel is a procedure that exfoliates injured or dead skin, enabling new skin to replace it. There are three types of chemical peels:

1. **Superficial:** This procedure removes the surface layer of the skin for a smoother, brighter appearance, and uses glycolic acid or dry ice for the peel.

2. **Medium:** This procedure is commonly used to smooth fine wrinkles, remove blemishes, and treat pigment problems. It uses trichloroacetic acid (TCA) for the peel.
3. **Deep:** This procedure is commonly used to correct coarse wrinkles and blotches on the face only and uses phenol for the peel. New skin might be lighter in tone because the skin loses some ability the produce pigment.

A chemical peel might change the patient's skin tone and result in scarring and cold sores. It might cause flaking and dryness.

20.3 Allergy Skin Test

An allergy skin test is performed to identify the source of a patient's allergic reaction.

Understanding the Allergy Skin Test

An allergen is a substance that causes an immune reaction. Allergy skin testing is performed to identify allergens. There are three types of skin testing for allergens:

1. **Skin Patch Test:** This test is used to identify allergens that cause contact dermatitis and requires the placement of a pad that contains an allergen solution on the skin for 72 hours. An allergic reaction occurs if the patient is allergic to the allergen.
2. **Skin Prick Test:** This test requires that a drop of an allergen solution be placed on the patient's skin. The skin is scratched, allowing the allergen solution to penetrate the skin. A wheal occurs if the patient is allergic to the allergen.
3. **Intradermal Test:** This test requires that a small amount of an allergen solution be injected into the dermal layer of the skin. A wheal occurs if the patient is allergic to the allergen.

20.4 Dermabrasion

Dermabrasion is performed to remove scars or growths from the upper layer of the skin and to remove wrinkles.

Understanding Dermabrasion

Dermabrasion is a procedure that removes the upper layers of damaged skin caused by scars and aging to encourage new skin growth. The procedure is performed by using a rotating burr to remove damaged tissue.

20.5 Mantoux Skin Test

The Mantoux skin test is performed to identify if the patient is or was ever exposed to *Mycobacterium tuberculosis*.

Understanding the Mantoux Skin Test

The Mantoux skin test determines if the patient has ever been exposed to *M. tuberculosis*. The health care provider injects the purified protein derivative (PPD), which is the *M. tuberculosis* antigen, into the patient's forearm. If the patient develops a wheal within 48 hours, indicating a positive immune response, then the patient either is or had been infected with *M. tuberculosis*. However, a positive Mantoux skin test doesn't always indicate that the patient has or had tuberculosis. Some patients may have received a tuberculosis vaccination that causes a positive result. A chest X-ray is taken to diagnose a current infection of *M. tuberculosis* should there be a positive immune response to the test.

20.6 Wound Culture

A wound culture is ordered to assess the existence and type of microorganism that is causing a skin infection. It is also used to assess which medication to use to treat the skin infection.

Understanding the Wound Culture Test

A wound culture is ordered when the patient is suspected of having a skin infection. A tissue sample of the infected area is taken and placed in an environment conducive to the growth of microorganisms for 3 days. The tissue sample is then examined to identify the presence and type of microorganism. Once the microorganism is identified, a sensitivity test is usually performed to determine the medication that kills the microorganism.

Solved Problems

Skin Tests

20.1 Why might a chemical peel be ordered?

A chemical peel is performed to cosmetically improve the patient's skin.

20.2 How does a chemical peel work?

A chemical peel is a procedure that exfoliates injured or dead skin, enabling new skin to replace it.

20.3 What is a superficial chemical peel?

This procedure removes the surface layer of the skin for a smoother, brighter appearance, and uses glycolic acid or dry ice for the peel.

20.4 What is a medium chemical peel?

This procedure is commonly used to smooth fine wrinkles, remove blemishes, and treat pigment problems.

20.5 What is a deep chemical peel?

This procedure is commonly used to correct coarse wrinkles and blotches on the face only.

20.6 Why might a health care provider use glycolic acid?

Glycolic acid is used for a superficial chemical peel.

20.7 When would a health care provider use phenol?

Phenol is used for a deep chemical peel.

20.8 What is a risk of performing a chemical peel?

A chemical peel might change the patient's skin tone and result in scarring and cold sores. It might cause flaking and dryness.

20.9 Why might a patient's new skin following a deep chemical peel have a lighter tone than the patient's normal skin?

New skin might be lighter in tone because the skin loses some ability to produce pigment.

20.10 Why might the health care provider use trichloroacetic acid (TCA)?

TCA is used for a medium chemical peel.

20.11 Why might a health care provider order an allergy skin test?

An allergy skin test is performed to identify the source of a patient's allergic reaction.

20.12 What is an allergen?

An allergen is a substance that causes an immune reaction.

20.13 What is a skin patch test?

This test is used to identify allergens that cause contact dermatitis and requires the placement of a pad that contains an allergen solution on the skin for 72 hours. An allergic reaction occurs if the patient is allergic to the allergen.

20.14 What is a skin prick test?

This test requires that a drop of an allergen solution be placed on the patient's skin. The skin is scratched, allowing the allergen solution to penetrate the skin.

20.15 How do you know if the skin prick test is positive?

A wheal occurs if the patient is allergic to the allergen.

20.16 What is an intradermal test?

This test requires that a small amount of an allergen solution be injected into the dermal layer of the skin.

20.17 Why is dermabrasion performed?

Dermabrasion is performed to remove scars and growths from the upper layer of the skin and to remove wrinkles.

20.18 How is dermabrasion performed?

The procedure is performed by using a rotating burr to remove damaged tissue.

20.19 Why is the Mantoux skin test ordered?

The Mantoux skin test is used to determine if the patient has or was exposed to *Mycobacterium tuberculosis*.

20.20 What is the purified protein derivative (PPD)?

The PPD is the *M. tuberculosis* antigen.

20.21 Where is the PPD injected?

The PPD is injected into the patient's forearm.

20.22 How do you determine if the Mantoux skin test is positive?

If the patient develops a wheal within 48 hours, indicating a positive immune response, then the patient either is or had been infected with *M. tuberculosis*.

20.23 Does a positive Mantoux skin test mean that the patient has or had tuberculosis?

No. Some patients may have received a tuberculosis vaccination that causes a positive result.

20.24 What might the health care provider do if the patient has a positive Mantoux skin test?

A chest X-ray is taken to diagnose a current infection of *M. tuberculosis* should there be a positive immune response to the test.

20.25 Why is a wound culture ordered?

A wound culture is ordered to assess the existence and type of a microorganism that is causing a skin infection. It is also used to assess which medication to use to treat the skin infection.

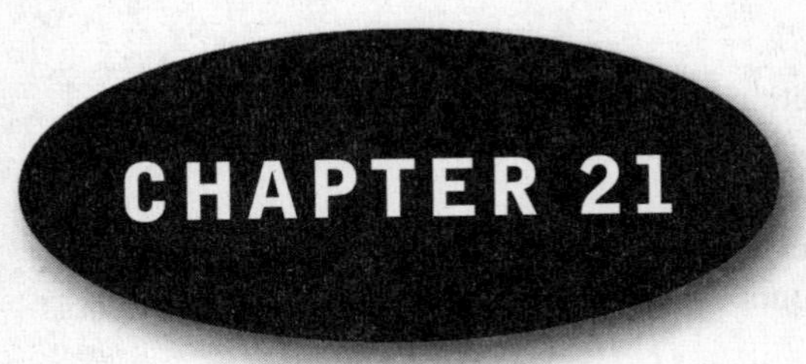

Foot Tests

21.1 Definition

There are a number of injuries and types of infection that affect the feet. The most common of these are bunions, a torn or ruptured Achilles tendon, or an injury or infection to a nail. A *bunion* is án abnormal alignment of the great toe that is characteristized by a protruding metatarsal joint and the great toe overlapping the neighboring toe. The *Achilles tendon* is the common term used for the *calcaneal tendon* that connects the heel of the foot to the calf. Contraction of the calcaneal tendon causes the foot to push down. Overuse of pushing down the foot might lead to inflammation. Injury might lead to a torn or ruptured calcaneal tendon. Nails can become injured or infected to a degree when all or a portion of the nail needs to be removed, allowing a new healthy nail to grow in its place.

21.2 Bunion Surgery

Bunion surgery is designed to provide relief of discomfort to the patient when standing or walking.

Understanding Bunion Surgery

Patients who have hallux valgus (abnormal angulation of the great toe) or hallux abductus valgus (abnormal inward leading of the great toe), which is commonly referred to as a bunion, can have the condition repaired by surgery. This condition is caused by pressure, resulting in malfunction of the tendons, ligaments, and structures that support the first metatarsal as a result of excessive ligamentous flexibility, abnormal bone growth, or flat feet. There is a genetic relationship with hallux valgus. The most common methods used to repair a bunion are:

- **Realignment:** This procedure realigns ligaments of the great toe joint.
- **Arthrodesis:** This procedure fuses the great toe joint.
- **Lapidus Procedure:** This procedure fuses the joint between the metatarsal bone joints and the mid foot.
- **Osteotomy:** This procedure removes a wedge from the foot or the great toe.
- **Bunionectomy:** This procedure removes the metatarsal head, which is the bone that bulges.
- **Implantation:** This procedure replaces the joint of the great toe with an artificial joint.
- **Resection Arthroplasty:** This procedure removes the bone from the end of the first metatarsal bone at the metatarsophalangeal joint and reshapes the great toe and the metatarsal bones.

21.3 Achilles Tendon Repair

The purpose of Achilles tendon repair is to restore movement to a foot.

Understanding Achilles Tendon Repair

The calcaneal tendon, commonly referred to as the Achilles tendon, connects the calf to the heel and can rupture or disconnect as result of injury. The Achilles tendon repair reconnects the tendon. There are two methods used to repair the Achilles tendon:

1. **Percutaneous Surgery:** This procedure reconnects the tendon through two or more small incisions.
2. **Open Surgery:** This procedure reconnects the tendon through a large incision.

21.4 Nail Removal

Nail removal is performed to remove an injured or infected nail.

Understanding Nail Removal

A health care provider removes all or part of a nail because of injury or due to a severe fungal infection, which is the most common nail infection. There are two methods of removing a nail:

1. **Debridement:** This procedure removes the part of nail that is damaged or infected.
2. **Avulsion:** This procedure removes the entire nail.

Solved Problems

Foot Tests

21.1 What is the Achilles tendon?

The Achilles tendon is the common term used for the calcaneal tendon that connects the heel of the foot to the calf.

21.2 What happens when the calcaneal tendon contracts?

Contraction of the calcaneal tendon causes the foot to push down.

21.3 What might occur if the calcaneal tendon is overly used?

Overuse of pushing down the foot might lead to inflammation.

21.4 What is a bunion?

A bunion is an abnormal alignment of the great toe that is characteristized by a protruding metatarsal joint and the great toe overlapping the neighboring toe.

21.5 What is the purpose of bunion surgery?

Bunion surgery is designed to provide relief of discomfort to the patient when standing or walking.

21.6 What is hallux valgus?

Hallux valgus is abnormal angulation of the great toe.

21.7 What is hallux abductus valgus?

Hallux abductus valgus is abnormal inward leading of the great toe.

21.8 What causes a bunion?

A bunion is caused by pressure resulting in malfunction of the tendons, ligaments, and structures that support the first metatarsal as a result of excessive ligamentous flexibility, abnormal bone growth, or flat feet.

21.9 What is realignment?

This procedure realigns ligaments of the great toe joint.

21.10 What is arthrodesis?

Arthrodesis fuses the great toe joint.

21.11 What is a Lapidus procedure?

The Lapidus procedure fuses the joint between the metatarsal bone joints and the mid-foot.

21.12 What is an osteotomy?

This procedure removes a wedge from the foot or the great toe.

21.13 What is a bunionectomy?

This procedure removes the metatarsal head, which is the bone that bulges.

21.14 What is an implantation?

Implantation replaces the joint of the great toe with an artificial joint.

21.15 What is resection arthroplasty?

Resection arthroplasty removes the bone from the end of the first metatarsal bone at the metatarsophalangeal joint and reshapes the great toe and the metatarsal bones.

21.16 What is the purpose of Achilles tendon repair?

The purpose of Achilles tendon repair is to restore movement to a foot.

21.17 What is a ruptured Achilles tendon?

The calcaneal tendon that connects the calf to the heel becomes disconnected.

21.18 What is percutaneous surgery?

Percutaneous surgery reconnects the tendon through two or more small incisions.

21.19 What is open surgery?

Open surgery reconnects the tendon through a large incision.

21.20 What is the most common nail infection?

A fungal infection is the most common nail infection.

21.21 What is debridement?

Debridement removes the part of nail that is damaged or infected.

21.22 What is avulsion?

Avulsion removes the entire nail.

21.23 What is a tendon?

A tendon is a band of fibrous connective tissue that connects muscle to bone.

21.24 What is a ligament?

A ligament is a band of connective tissue that connects together two or more bones or cartilages.

21.25 What is the metatarsophalangeal joint?

The metatarsophalangeal joint is the joint closest to the foot that connects the toe to the foot.

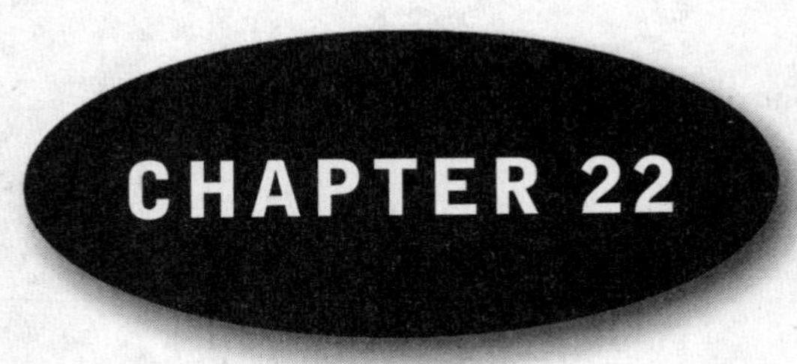

Vision Tests and Procedures

22.1 Definition

Light rays pass through the cornea, the pupil, and lenses, which focus the ray of light onto the retina located at the back of the eye. When light rays are not properly focused on the retina, the patient is unable to see clearly.

Light rays focused in front of the retina causes *myopia* (nearsightedness), enabling patients to better see things near them than at a distance. Light rays focused behind the retina causes *hyperopia* (farsightedness), enabling patients to see things at a distance better than up close. When light rays are irregularly bent, images are blurred, resulting in *astigmatism*.

A standard vision test is used to assess the patient's ability to see close up and at a distance. It also determines if the patient is experiencing peripheral vision difficulty or might have macular degeneration. In addition, the test determines the refractive error of the patient's eye, which determines the corrective lenses needed to restore the patient's eyesight.

Patients who have myopia might be able to have this condition fixed by having corneal ring implants or by reshaping the cornea using photorefractive keratectomy.

A trabeculectomy or a trabeculotomy can be performed to drain aqueous humor that might be backing up because of a blockage in the trabecular meshwork. Seton glaucoma surgery might be performed to insert a drainage tube in the eye to drain the aqueous humor.

Blood flow in the eye can be assessed by performing an eye angiogram, which detects a *vitreous hemorrhage*. A vitreous hemorrhage is treated by performing a *vitrectomy*.

A detached retina occurs when the retina is detached from the back wall of the eye. When this occurs, the health care provider can repair the problem by performing a sclera buckling to relieve traction on the retina. A *pneumatic retinopexy* might be performed to push the retina back into position, using a gas bubble.

22.2 Vision Tests

Vision tests are performed to correct the patient's vision with glasses or contact lenses and to determine if the patient is color blind or losing peripheral vision, or to determine if the patient has macular degeneration. Vision tests determine the refractive error of the patient's eye, which determines the proper corrective lenses needed to restore the patient's eyesight.

Understanding Vision Tests

The health care provider examines the patient's peripheral vision and ability to see near and far distances along with the patient's ability to distinguish colors by performing nine vision tests:

1. **Confrontation:** This test assesses the patient's peripheral vision by gazing at the health care provider's nose.

2. **Amsler Grid:** This test assesses for macular degeneration.
3. **Perimetry:** This test assesses the patient's peripheral vision by flashing lights randomly in a perimeter.
4. **Tangent Screen:** This test assesses the patient's peripheral vision by gazing at a concentric circle image.
5. **Snellen:** This test assesses the patient's ability to see distances.
6. **E Chart:** This chart is used to assess the patient's ability to see distances when the patient is unable to read.
7. **Near:** This test assesses the patient's ability to see near distances.
8. **Color Vision:** This test assesses the patient's ability to distinguish colors.
9. **Refraction:** This test measures the refractive error of the patient's eyes to determine the lens that will correct the patient's eyesight.

22.3 Tonometry Test

The tonometry test is a test to screen for glaucoma.

Understanding the Tonometry Test

Tonometry measures the intraocular pressure of the patient's eye by assessing the amount of pressure necessary to flatten the cornea. There are four methods used to perform tonometry:

- **Pneumotonometry:** This method uses a puff of air to measure intraocular pressure. No direct contact is made with the eye.
- **Applanation:** This method uses a tonometer to measure intraocular pressure based on the force required to flatten (applanate) a constant area of the cornea.
- **Electronic Indentation:** This method uses a tonometer that is connected to a computer to measure intraocular pressure.
- **Schiotz:** This method uses a plunger to measure intraocular pressure.

22.4 Electronystagmogram (ENG)

Electronystagmogram (ENG) assesses the underlying cause of loss of balance and vertigo.

Understanding the Electronystagmogram

The electronystagmogram is a test that measures eye movement (both voluntary eye movement and nystagmus) to assess the patient's balance and the underlying cause of vertigo.

Solved Problems

Vision Tests and Procedures

22.1 What is a common reason for a patient to not see clearly?

Light rays pass through the cornea, the pupil, and lenses, which focus the ray of light onto the retina located at the back of the eye. When light rays are not properly focused on the retina, the patient is unable to see clearly.

22.2 What is myopia?

Light rays focused in front of the retina cause myopia (nearsightedness), enabling patients to better see things near them than at a distance.

22.3 What is hyperopia?

Light rays focused behind the retina cause hyperopia (farsightedness), enabling patients to see things at a distance better than up close.

22.4 What is astigmatism?

When light rays are irregularly bent, images are blurred, resulting in astigmatism.

22.5 What is a detached retina?

A detached retina occurs when the retina is detached from the back wall of the eye.

22.6 How might a health care provider repair a detached retina?

When a detached retina occurs, the health care provider can repair the problem by performing a sclera buckling to relieve traction on the retina. A pneumatic retinopexy might be performed to push the retina back into position, using a gas bubble.

22.7 Why are vision tests performed?

Vision tests are performed to correct the patient's vision with glasses or contact lenses and to determine if the patient is color blind or losing peripheral vision, or to determine if the patient has macular degeneration.

22.8 How does the health care provider know what corrective lenses are needed to restore the patient's eyesight?

Vision tests determine the refractive error of the patient's eye, which determines the proper corrective lenses needed to restore the patient's eye sight.

22.9 What is a confrontation test?

A confrontation test assesses the patient's peripheral vision by gazing at the health care provider's nose.

22.10 What is the Amsler grid test?

The Amsler grid test assesses for macular degeneration.

22.11 What is a perimetry test?

A perimetry test assesses the patient's peripheral vision by flashing lights randomly in a perimeter.

22.12 What is the tangent screen test?

The tangent screen test assesses the patient's peripheral vision by gazing at a concentric circle image.

22.13 What is a Snellen test?

A Snellen test assesses the patient's ability to see distances.

22.14 What is the E chart?

The E chart assesses the patient's ability to see distances when the patient is unable to read.

22.15 What is the near test?

The near test assesses the patient's ability to see near distances.

22.16 What is the color vision test?

The color vision test assesses the patient's ability to distinguish colors.

22.17 What is the refraction test?

The refraction test measures the refractive error of the patient's eyes to determine the lens that will correct the patient's eyesight.

22.18 Why is the tonometry test performed?

The tonometry test is performed to screen for glaucoma.

22.19 What is measured by the tonometry test?

The tonometry test measures the intraocular pressure of the patient's eye.

22.20 What is pneumotonometry?

Pneumotonometry uses a puff of air to measure intraocular pressure. No direct contact is made with the eye.

22.21 What is applanation tonometry?

Applanation tonometry uses a tonometer to measure intraocular pressure based on the force required to flatten (applanate) a constant area of the cornea.

22.22 What is electronic indentation tonometry?

Electronic indentation tonometry uses a tonometer that is connected to a computer to measure intraocular pressure.

22.23 What is Schiotz tonometry?

Schiotz tonometry uses a plunger to measure intraocular pressure.

22.24 Why is an electronystagmogram (ENG) administered?

An ENG assesses the underlying cause of loss of balance and vertigo.

22.25 What is measured in an ENG?

An ENG is a test that measures both voluntary eye movement and nystagmus to assess the patient's balance and evaluate the underlying cause of vertigo.

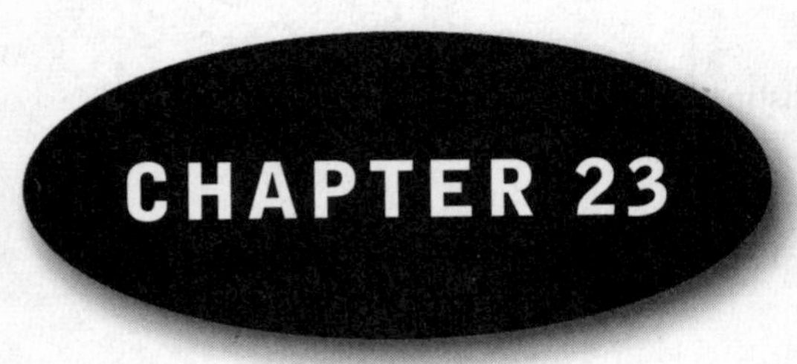

Cardiovascular Terminology

23.1 Definition

The cardiovascular system is responsible for delivery of blood, which carries oxygen and other nutrients to the tissues of the body. The heart pumps the blood to the body, where it delivers nutrients and oxygen, picks up waste products, and then returns to the heart.

The heart has four chambers. The upper chambers are the atria; the lower chambers are the ventricles. In the middle there is a septum, a wall that separates the right side of the heart from the left side of the heart. Atrioventricular (AV) valves control the blood flow between the upper and lower chambers of the heart.

The tricuspid valve is on the right side; the mitral valve is on the left side between the atria and the ventricle. The pulmonic valve controls the flow between the right ventricle and the pulmonary artery, whereas the aortic valve controls the flow between the left ventricle and the aorta.

Unoxygenated blood empties into the right atrium from the systemic circulation via the inferior vena cava and superior vena cava. As the right atrium contracts, the tricuspid valve opens, allowing the blood to flow into the right ventricle. With contraction of the right ventricle, the pulmonic valve opens, allowing the unoxygenated blood to enter the pulmonary artery to go to the lungs to pick up oxygen.

Once oxygenated, the blood returns to the heart via the pulmonary vein and enters the left atrium. As the left atrium contracts, the mitral valve opens, allowing the blood to flow into the left ventricle. As the left ventricle contracts, the aortic valve opens, allowing the blood to flow into the aorta and systemic circulation. The blood returns to the heart from the lower body via the inferior vena cava and from the upper body via the superior vena cava. The functions on the right side and left side of the heart happen simultaneously.

Therefore, when we listen to a normal heartbeat, the sounds we hear are the sounds of the valves closing. The mitral and tricuspid valves create the first heart sound (S_1), whereas aortic and pulmonic valves create the second heart sound (S_2).

The electrical conduction system of the heart starts at the sinoatrial (SA) node, which is located in the right atrium. It initiates the heart beat, ranging from 60 to 100 beats per minute, every day, for a lifetime.

The electrical current travels across both atria, then converges on the AV node where the current slows, allowing the atria to repolarize. The AV node is located in the superior portion of the ventricular septum. In the bottom portion are located the right and left bundle of His, which is a group of special cardiac muscles that send an electrical impulse to the ventricle to begin cardiac contractions.

These end in the Purkinje fibers and spread out through the ventricles. The current passing through these fibers causes ventricular contraction, forcing the blood from the right ventricle to the lungs, and the left ventricle to the aorta, thus creating systemic circulation.

23.2 Aortic Aneurysm

A weakening in the wall of a portion of the aorta results in a balloon-like bulge as blood flows through the aorta. The blood flow within this bulging area of the aorta becomes very turbulent. Over time, this turbulence can cause the dilated area to increase in size, creating an aneurysm. The aneurysm can rupture, causing a disruption in blood flow to everything below the affected area, and may even result in death.

This is commonly caused by atherosclerosis, in which fatty substances, cholesterol, calcium, and the clotting material fibrin (referred to as plaque), buildup in the inner lining of an artery and result in thickening and hardening of the arteries. It may also be caused by degeneration of the smooth muscle layer (middle) of the aorta, trauma, congenital defect, or infection. The aneurysm may be found incidentally on radiographic studies done for other reasons, or the patient may have developed symptoms indicating that something was wrong, such as severe back or abdominal pain, or a pulsating mass. Severe hypotension and syncope (fainting caused by insufficient blood supply to the brain) may indicate rupture.

23.3 Angina (Angina Pectoris)

A narrowing of blood vessels to the coronary artery, secondary to arteriosclerosis, results in inadequate blood flow through blood vessels of the heart muscle, causing chest pain. An episode of angina is typically precipitated by physical activity, excitement, or emotional stress. There are three categories of angina:

- **Stable:** The pain is relieved by rest or nitrates and symptoms are consistent.
- **Unstable:** The pain occurs at rest; is of new onset; is of increasing intensity, force, or duration; is not relieved by rest; and is slow to subside in response to nitroglycerin.
- **Prinzmetal's or Vasospastic:** This usually occurs at rest or with minimal formal exercise or exertion; it often occurs at night.

Atherosclerotic heart disease occurs when there is a buildup of plaque within the coronary arteries. Angina is often the first symptom that heart disease exists. When the demand for oxygen by the heart muscle exceeds the available supply, chest pain occurs.

23.4 Myocardial Infarction (MI)

Blood supply to the myocardium is interrupted for a prolonged time because of the blockage of coronary arteries. This results in insufficient oxygen reaching cardiac muscle, causing cardiac muscles to die (necrosis). Myocardial infarction is commonly known as a heart attack. The area of infarction is often due to a buildup of plaque over time (atherosclerosis). It may also be caused by a clot that develops in association with the atherosclerosis within the vessel. Patients are typically (but not always) symptomatic. However, some patients are not aware of the event; they have what is called a silent MI.

23.5 Coronary Artery Disease (CAD)

Cholesterol, calcium, and other elements carried by the blood are deposited on the wall of the coronary artery, resulting in the narrowing of the artery and the reduction of blood flow through the vessel. This impedes blood supply to the heart muscle. These deposits start out as fatty streaks and eventually develop into plaque that inhibits blood flow through the artery. Elevated cholesterol levels and fat intake can contribute to this plaque buildup, as can hypertension, diabetes, and smoking. When the plaque builds up within the artery, the heart muscle is deprived of oxygen and nutrients, ultimately damaging the heart muscle.

23.6 Peripheral Arterial Disease (PAD)

Large peripheral arteries become narrowed and restricted (stenosis), leading to the temporary (acute) or permanent (chronic) reduction of blood flow to tissues (ischemia). This is most commonly caused by atherosclerosis (plaque on the inner walls of arteries), but may also be caused by a blood clot (embolism), or an inflammatory process. Severe peripheral arterial occlusive disease can lead to skin ulceration and gangrene. Peripheral arterial occlusive disease is more common in patients with diabetes or hypertension, older adults, those with hyperlipidemia, and those who smoke, as these conditions can predispose the patient to diminished circulation. Vascular disease that happens in one area of the body (i.e., coronary arteries) is not an isolated process. The plaque buildup caused by long-term elevated cholesterol levels happens throughout the body. The most common area of involvement is the lower extremities.

23.7 Cardiac Tamponade

A large amount of liquid accumulates in the sack around the heart (pericardium), creating pressure on the heart that reduces the filling of ventricles with blood. This results in a low volume of blood being pumped with each contraction. The accumulating pressure within the pericardium may result from fluid, pus, or blood. The end result is decreased stroke volume and cardiac output. The cause of tamponade may be trauma, postoperative, post-MI, uremia, or cancer. The fluid may develop rapidly or over time, depending on the cause. Tamponade is a life-threatening condition. The seriousness is related to the amount of pressure within the heart and the resulting decrease in ventricular filling.

23.8 Cardiogenic Shock

Cardiogenic shock is caused by a drop in blood pressure and blood flow caused by the heart's inability to pump blood as a result of a cardiac emergency such as cardiac tamponade, myocardial ischemia, myocarditis, or cardiomyo-pathy (a disease of the heart that deteriorates the heart function). Blood pools in the left ventricle, which causes a backup of blood into the lungs, resulting in pulmonary edema. Contractions increase to compensate for the decreased cardiac output causing an increase in demand for oxygen by the heart. However, the lungs are not oxygenating the blood sufficiently because of decreased blood flow; therefore, heart muscles are starved for oxygen.

23.9 Cardiomyopathy

The middle layer of the heart wall that contains cardiac muscle (myocardium) weakens and stretches, causing the heart to lose its pumping strength and become enlarged. The heart remains functional; however, contractions are weak, resulting in decreased cardiac output. Most are idiopathic and not related to the major causes of heart disease.

The three types of cardiomyopathy are:

- **Dilated (Common):** The heart muscle thins and enlarges, which leads to congestive heart failure. Progressive hypertrophy and dilatation result in problems with pumping action of ventricles.
- **Hypertrophic:** The ventricular heart muscle thickens, resulting in outflow obstruction or restriction. There is some blood flow present.
- **Restrictive (Rare):** The heart muscle becomes stiff and restricts blood from filling ventricles, usually as a result of amyloidosis, radiation, or myocardial fibrosis after open heart surgery.

23.10 Endocarditis

Microorganisms, usually bacteria, enter the bloodstream and attach to the inner lining of the heart (endocardium) and heart valves, resulting in inflammation. Ulceration and necrosis occur when microorganisms cover the heart valves. This usually occurs in patients with rheumatic or degenerative heart disease; those with recent instrumentation [IV, genitourinary (GU), and respiratory procedures] or dental procedures; and IV drug users.

23.11 Heart Failure [Congestive Heart Failure (CHF)]

In congestive heart failure (CHF), the heart is unable to pump sufficient blood to maintain adequate circulation. This result in a backup of blood and the extra pressure may cause accumulation of fluid. Heart failure is primarily caused by problems with ventricular pumping action of the cardiac muscle, which may be caused by diseases such as MI (heart attack), endocarditis (infection in the heart), hypertension (high blood pressure), or valvular insufficiency. When disease affects primarily the left side of the heart, the blood backs up into the lungs. When disease affects primarily the right side of the heart, systemic circulation may be overloaded. When the heart failure becomes significant, the whole circulatory system may become compromised.

23.12 Hypertension

Pressure inside blood vessels exceeds 140 mm Hg systolic and 90 mm Hg diastolic on more than one occasion resulting from a primary disease or no known cause. These are the classifications of hypertension:

- **Normal:** <120 mm Hg systolic / <80 mm Hg diastolic
- **Prehypertension:** 120–139 mm Hg systolic / 80–89 mm Hg diastolic
- **Stage 1:** 140–159 mm Hg systolic / 90–99 mm Hg diastolic
- **Stage 2:** 160 mm Hg systolic / 100 mm Hg diastolic
- **Diabetes Hypertension:** >130 mm Hg systolic / >80 mm Hg diastolic

23.13 Hypovolemic Shock

Rapid fluid loss causes inadequate circulation, resulting in inadequate perfusion of organs. Hypovolemic shock can be caused by external hemorrhage, fluids moving in the body from vessels into tissue (third spacing), or dehydration. External hemorrhage is loss of blood, plasma, fluids, and electrolytes because of trauma, gastrointestinal bleed, vomiting, or diarrhea. Third spacing can result from ascites or pancreatitis.

23.14 Myocarditis

Inflammation of the heart muscle is usually caused by infection, most often viral. Infection can also be caused by alcohol poisoning from chronic alcohol abuse, drugs, or diseases that can result in the degeneration of heart muscle. This reduces the ability of the heart to pump blood efficiently, leading to CHF.

23.15 Pericarditis

The membrane that encloses the heart (pericardium) is inflamed. Pericarditis is either acute or chronic. Acute pericarditis is most commonly associated with viral infections. Upper respiratory symptoms are not uncommon and can occur a few weeks before the onset of pericarditis. Pericarditis may be caused by any infectious agent, acute myocardial infarction (AMI), malignancy, autoimmune diseases, or drug reaction.

23.16 Pulmonary Edema

Fluid builds up in the lungs from ineffective pumping of blood by the heart as a result of left-sided heart failure, AMI, worsening of heart failure, or volume overload. The patient experiences hypoxia, which is insufficient oxygen supply to tissues, caused by decreased oxygenation of the blood. Several noncardiac issues may lead to pulmonary embolism.

23.17 Raynaud's Disease

Blood flow to the extremities decreases as peripheral arteries narrow from vasospasm when exposed to cold or emotional stress. This results in the fingers, toes, nose, and ears blanching to a pale shade and/or turning blue and red as blood flow decreases. It usually occurs bilaterally, often sparing the thumbs, and begins to resolve with warming of affected areas. Raynaud's is a benign condition usually controlled by avoidance of underlying factors (i.e., cold and stress). Secondary Raynaud's can be seen with other disorders, mostly inflammatory and/or connective tissue diseases. This is more common in older men, usually involves the hands, and can have other complications.

23.18 Rheumatic Heart Disease

Rheumatic fever usually results from a prior upper respiratory infection with group A streptococcus. It may lead to permanent valve disease and cardiac damage, with the mitral valve being more commonly affected.

23.19 Thrombophlebitis

Thrombophlebitis is the inflammation of a vein as a result of the formation of one or more blood clots (thrombus). It is usually seen in the lower extremities, calves, or pelvis. This may be the result of injury to the area, may be precipitated by certain medications or poor blood flow, or may be the result of a coagulation disorder.

23.20 Atrial Fibrillation

Uncoordinated firing of electrical impulses in the wall of the atria (upper chambers of the heart) causes the heart to quiver instead of beat regularly, resulting in ineffective contractions. This is usually caused by an abnormality in the electrical system of the heart. Blood is ineffectively pumped to the ventricles (lower chambers of the heart) and may result in not enough blood being pumped throughout the body. Usually the heart beats rapidly; however, this is not always the case. Atrial fibrillation (also called AF or "a fib") is the most common chronic arrhythmia and is not life threatening on its own, but increases the patient's risk for blood clots and strokes.

23.21 Asystole

Asystole is defined as no cardiac electrical activity. This causes ventricles to stop contractions, leading to no cardiac output and no blood flow. Cardiac standstill is a medical emergency. Treatment must be started immediately, while simultaneously attempting to understand the etiology of a nonbeating heart. Asystole is a criterion for certifying that the patient is dead. Asystole may be caused by disruption in the electrical conduction system, causing life-threatening arrhythmias, sudden cardiac death, hypovolemia, cardiac tamponade, massive pulmonary embolism, AMI, metabolic disorder, or drug overdoses. In case of a drug overdose—usually PEA (pulseless electrical activity)—reverse overdose or treat.

23.22 Ventricular Fibrillation

Electrical impulses that trigger the ventricles to contract fire erratically. This causes the ventricles to quiver and prevents regular effective contractions, resulting in the disruption of blood flow to the body. The usual causes are ventricular tachycardia, electrolyte disturbances, MI, electric shock, and drug toxicities.

23.23 Ventricular Tachycardia

Abnormal electrical impulses within the ventricles cause the heart to contract more than 160 beats per minute. This results in inadequate filling of the ventricles with blood between beats; subsequently, less blood is pumped throughout the body than during normal contractions. Ventricular tachycardia (called "V tach") often occurs after AMI and in cardiomyopathy, coronary artery disease (CAD), mitral valve prolapse, and other myocardial disease.

23.24 Aortic Insufficiency (AI)

Leakage of the aortic valve causes blood to flow back into the left ventricle. This results in increased blood volume in the left ventricle, causing it to dilate and become hypertrophic, thus reducing blood flow from the heart. The usual cause is incompetent cusps or leaflets of the valve, from endocarditis, valve structural problems, connective tissue disorders, rheumatic heart disease, hypertension, arteriosclerosis, and other conditions.

23.25 Mitral Insufficiency

Leakage of the mitral valve causes blood to flow back from the left ventricle into the left atrium. As a result, blood might flow back into the lungs. Mitral regurgitation is caused by an incompetent valve, damaged from rheumatic fever, CAD, or endocarditis.

23.26 Mitral Stenosis

In mitral stenosis, scar tissue secondary to rheumatic fever forms on the mitral valve. This causes it to narrow, increasing resistance to blood flow between the left ventricle and left atrium, which means the heart needs to pump harder to maintain blood flow.

23.27 Mitral Valve Prolapse

The mitral valve bulges back into the left atrium, allowing blood to flow backward from the left ventricle into the left atrium. This is a common problem and is not considered a serious condition. It is often congenital.

23.28 Tricuspid Insufficiency

Leakage in the tricuspid valve causes a backflow from the right ventricle into the right atrium. This results in increased pressure in the atrium and higher resistance to blood flowing from veins, causing enlargement of the right atrium. This may occur from an anatomic problem, but usually occurs from right ventricular overload (in turn caused by left ventricular overload). It may also occur because of an inferior MI, or damage from endocarditis.

23.29 Cardiac Catheterization (Angiography)

This is an invasive procedure used to examine the coronary arteries and intracardiac structures, as well as to measure cardiac output, intracardiac pressures, and oxygenation.

A radiopaque dye, which makes structures visible on X-rays, is injected through a catheter into the femoral artery in the patient's left leg or in the antecubital fossa, which is the crease of the arm; it then flows to the coronary arteries. The flow of the radiopaque dye is viewed and recorded using a fluoroscope, enabling the health care provider to determine obstructions to the flow and the structures of the heart.

23.30 Echocardiograph

An ultrasound of the heart provides a noninvasive examination of intracardiac structures and blood flow. Sound waves are directed to and deflected by the heart, causing an echo that is detected by the echocardiograph, which is interpreted by a health care provider.

23.31 Nuclear Cardiology

These tests determine myocardial perfusion and contractility of the heart, ischemia, infarction, wall motion, and ejection fraction. Radioisotopes are injected through the IV. The radiation detector monitors the flow of the radioisotope as it flows through the heart.

23.32 Digital Subtraction Angiography

Digital subtraction angiography enables the health care provider to view arterial blood supply to the heart using an injection of radiopaque contrast material. The patient is injected with an intravascular contrast material containing iodine. Images of bone and soft tissue are viewed from fluoroscopy through the use of a computer, enabling the health care provider to view the cardiovascular system.

23.33 Hemodynamic Monitoring

Hemodynamic monitoring measures cardiac output and intracardiac pressure. A balloon-tipped catheter is inserted into the pulmonary artery, usually through the femoral artery. It is able to measure pressures in the heart's various chambers and vessels.

23.34 Venogram

This determines if the patient has incomplete valves or deep vein thrombosis. An iodine dye is injected into the vein, making the vein visible in a fluoroscope; this allows the health care provider to visualize the flow of venous blood.

23.35 Pulse Oximetry

This determines the abbreviated arterial oxygen saturation of the blood. The full arterial oxygen saturation is determined by the arterial blood gas test.

An infrared light passes through the patient's nailbed or skin. The amount of infrared light passing through determines the amount of arterial oxygen saturation of the blood.

Solved Problems

Cardiovascular Terminology

23.1 What is an aortic aneurysm?

An aortic aneurysm is a weakening in the wall of a portion of the aorta resulting in a balloon-like bulge as blood flows through the aorta.

23.2 What is a common cause of an aortic aneurysm?

An aortic aneurysm is commonly caused by atherosclerosis, in which fatty substances, cholesterol, calcium, and the clotting material fibrin, referred to as plaque, buildup in the inner lining of an artery, resulting in thickening and hardening of the arteries.

23.3 What is angina pectoris?

Angina pectoris is a narrowing of blood vessels to the coronary artery, secondary to arteriosclerosis, resulting in inadequate blood flow through blood vessels of the heart muscle, causing chest pain.

23.4 What is Prinzmetal's angina?

Prinzmetal's angina usually occurs at rest or with minimal formal exercise or exertion; it often occurs at night.

23.5 What is a myocardial infarction (MI)?

Blood supply to the myocardium is interrupted for a prolonged time because of the blockage of coronary arteries. This results in insufficient oxygen reaching cardiac muscle, causing cardiac muscles to die (necrosis). Myocardial infarction is commonly known as a heart attack.

23.6 What is peripheral arterial disease (PAD)?

Large peripheral arteries become narrowed and restricted (stenosis), leading to the temporary (acute) or permanent (chronic) reduction of blood flow to tissues (ischemia). This is most commonly caused by atherosclerosis (plaque on the inner walls of arteries), but may also be caused by a blood clot (embolism), or an inflammatory process.

23.7 What is cardiac tamponade?

A large amount of liquid accumulates in the sack around the heart (pericardium), creating pressure on the heart that reduces the filling of ventricles with blood.

23.8 What is a common cause of cardiac tamponade?

The accumulating pressure within the pericardium may result from fluid, pus, or blood.

23.9 What is the result of cardiac tamponade?

Cardiac tamponade results in a low volume of blood being pumped with each contraction. The end result is decreased stroke volume and cardiac output.

23.10 What is cardiogenic shock?

Cardiogenic shock is a drop in blood pressure and blood flow caused by the heart's inability to pump blood as a result of a cardiac emergency.

23.11 What are common causes of cardiogenic shock?

Common causes of cardiogenic shock are cardiac tamponade, myocardial ischemia, myocarditis, or cardiomyopathy.

23.12 What is cardiomyopathy?

The middle layer of the heart wall that contains cardiac muscle (myocardium) weakens and stretches, causing the heart to lose its pumping strength and become enlarged.

23.13 What is a common result of cardiomyopathy?

The heart remains functional; however, contractions are weak, resulting in decreased cardiac output.

23.14 What is hypertrophic cardiomyopathy?

The ventricular heart muscle thickens, resulting in outflow obstruction or restriction. There is some blood flow present.

23.15 What is endocarditis?

Microorganisms, usually bacteria, enter the bloodstream and attach to the inner lining of the heart (endocardium) and heart valves, resulting in inflammation.

23.16 Why should a health care provider anticipate endocarditis developing?

This usually occurs in patients with rheumatic heart disease or degenerative heart disease; those with recent instrumentation [IV, genitoutinary (GU), and respiratory procedures] or dental procedures; and IV drug users.

23.17 What is congestive heart failure (CHF)?

In CHF, the heart is unable to pump sufficient blood to maintain adequate circulation. This result in a backup of blood, and the extra pressure may cause accumulation of fluid.

23.18 What causes CHF?

Heart failure is primarily caused by problems with ventricular pumping action of the cardiac muscle, which may be caused by diseases such as MI (heart attack), endocarditis (infection in the heart), hypertension (high blood pressure), or valvular insufficiency.

23.19 When does fluid back up into the lungs in CHF?

When disease affects primarily the left side of the heart, the blood will back up into the lungs.

23.20 When does fluid back up into the circulation in CHF?

When disease affects primarily the right side of the heart, the systemic circulation may be overloaded.

23.21 What is hypovolemic shock?

Rapid fluid loss causes inadequate circulation, resulting in inadequate perfusion of organs.

23.22 What are common causes of hypovolemic shock?

Hypovolemic shock can be caused by external hemorrhage, fluids moving in the body from vessels into tissue (third spacing), or dehydration.

23.23 What is pericarditis?

Pericarditis occurs when the membrane that encloses the heart (pericardium) is inflamed.

23.24 What is Raynaud's disease?

Blood flow to the extremities decreases as peripheral arteries narrow from vasospasm when exposed to cold or emotional stress. This results in the fingers, toes, nose, and ears blanching to a pale shade and/or turning blue and red as blood flow decreases.

23.25 What is thrombophlebitis?

Thrombophlebitis is the inflammation of a vein as a result of the formation of one or more blood clots (thrombus).

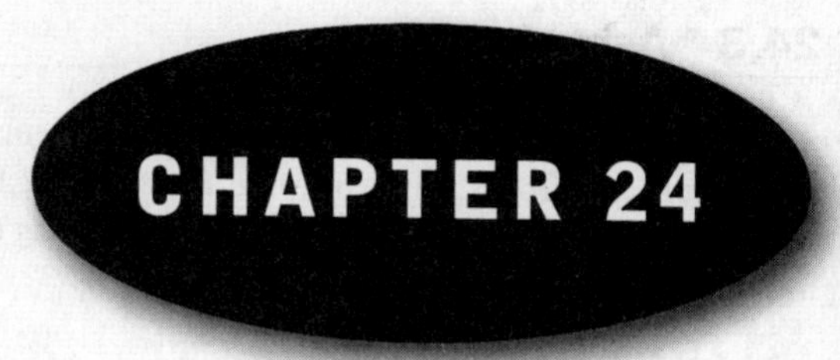

CHAPTER 24

The Respiratory System

24.1 Definition

The respiratory system has the following basic functions:

- Movement of air in and out of the lungs
- Exchange of oxygen and carbon dioxide
- Helping maintain acid-base balance

Ventilation moves air in (inspiration) and out (expiration) of the lungs. During inspiration, air flows in through the nose and passes into the nasopharynx. Air is then drawn through the pharynx, larynx, trachea, and bronchi. The bronchi branches (bifurcates) right and left into smaller tubes called bronchioles that terminate in alveoli.

The airways are lined with mucous membranes to add moisture to the inhaled air. There is a thin layer of mucus in the airways that helps to trap foreign particles such as dust, pollen, or bacteria. Cilia—small, hairlike projections—help to move the mucus with the foreign material upward so it can be coughed out.

Alveoli are air-filled sacs containing membranes coated with surfactant. The surfactant helps the alveoli to expand evenly on inspiration and prevents collapse on exhalation. Carbon dioxide and oxygen are exchanged; a higher concentration of gas moves to the lower area of concentration. A higher concentration of carbon dioxide in the hemoglobin moves across the membranes into the alveoli and is expired by the lungs. The higher concentration of oxygen in the alveoli crosses the membrane and attaches to the hemoglobin, which is then distributed by the circulatory system throughout the body.

Lungs are contained within a pleural sac in the thoracic cavity and operate on negative pressure. The visceral pleura is close to the lungs and the parietal pleura is close to the chest wall. There is a pleural space between these two layers that contains a small amount of fluid to prevent friction with chest movement on inspiration and expiration.

24.2 Acute Respiratory Distress Syndrome (ARDS)

Patients develop acute respiratory failure. Lungs stiffen as a result of a buildup of fluid in the lungs. Fluid builds up in the tissue of the lungs (interstitium) and the alveoli. This fluid and stiffness impairs the lungs' ability to move air in and out (ventilation). There is an inflammatory response in the tissues of the lungs.

Damage to the surfactant within the alveoli leads to alveolar collapse, further impairing gas exchange. An attempt to repair the alveolar damage may lead to fibrosis within the lung. Even as the respiratory rate increases, sufficient oxygen cannot get into the circulation (hypoxemia).

Oxygen saturation decreases. Respiratory acidosis develops, and the patient appears to have respiratory distress. This is most commonly caused by shock, sepsis, or as a result of trauma or inhalation injury. Patients may have no history of pulmonary disorders, also known as adult respiratory distress syndrome.

24.3 Asbestosis

Asbestos fibers enter the lungs, causing inflammation in the bronchioles and the walls of the alveoli. After inhalation, the fibers settle into the lung tissue. Fibrosis develops and ultimately pleural plaques form. The changes within the lung result in a restrictive lung disease. The damage to the lung causes impairment in breathing and air exchange.

24.4 Asthma

The airways become obstructed from either inflammation of the lining of the airways or constriction of the bronchial smooth muscles (bronchospasm). A known allergen (for example, pollen) is inhaled, causing activation of antibodies that recognize the allergen. Mast cells and histamine are activated, initiating a local inflammatory response. Prostaglandins enhance the effect of histamine.

Leukotrienes also respond, enhancing the inflammatory response. White blood cells responding to the area release inflammatory mediators. A stimulus causes an inflammatory reaction, increasing the size of the bronchial linings; this results in restriction of the airways. There may be a bronchial smooth muscle reaction at the same time.

There are two kinds of asthma:

- **Extrinsic:** Also known as atopic, caused by allergens such as pollen, animal dander, mold, or dust. Often accompanied by allergic rhinitis and eczema; this may run in families.
- **Intrinsic:** Also known as nonatopic, caused by a nonallergic factor such as following a respiratory tract infection, exposure to cold air, changes in air humidity, or respiratory irritants.

24.5 Atelectasis

A portion of the lung does not expand completely, decreasing the lung's capacity to exchange gases and resulting in decreased oxygenation of blood. Obstruction of part of the airway causes collapse distal to the area that is blocked. Obstruction can be from a mucous plug inside the airway, or a tumor or fluid within the pleural space that may be pressing on the airway from the outside. Postoperatively, patients are at risk for atelectasis because of pain, immobility, medications for pain, anesthesia, and lack of deep breathing.

24.6 Bronchiectasis

Bronchi and bronchioles become abnormally and permanently dilated because of infection and inflammation. This results in excessive production of mucus that obstructs the bronchi. There is some obstruction of the airways and a chronic infection. The changes within the lung can be localized or generalized. The lung may develop areas of atelectasis where thick mucus obstructs the smaller airways, making the mucus difficult to expel. This results in inflammation and infection of the airways and leads to bronchitis.

24.7 Bronchitis

Increased mucus production, caused by infection and airborne irritants that block airways in the lungs, results in the decreased ability to exchange gases. There are two forms of bronchitis: acute, in which blockage of the airways is reversible; and chronic, in which blockage is not reversible.

Patients with acute bronchitis are symptomatic typically for 7 to 10 days, often because of viral (but sometimes bacterial) infection. Patients with chronic bronchitis have symptoms of a chronic productive cough for at least 3 consecutive months and up to 2 consecutive years. There is increased mucus production, inflammatory changes, and, ultimately, fibrosis in the airway walls. The patient with chronic bronchitis has an increased incidence of respiratory infection.

24.8 Cor Pulmonale

In cor pulmonale, the structure and function of the right ventricle are compromised by chronic obstructive pulmonary disease (COPD), obstruction of the airflow into and out of the lungs. The heart tries to compensate, resulting in right-sided heart failure. The patient has heart failure because of a primary lung disorder that causes pulmonary hypertension and enlargement of the right ventricle. Patients have symptoms of both the underlying pulmonary disorder and the right-sided heart failure. COPD consists of chronic bronchitis and emphysema.

24.9 Emphysema

Chronic inflammation reduces the flexibility of the walls of the alveoli, resulting in overdistention of the alveolar walls. This causes air to be trapped in the lungs, impeding gas exchange. Smoking is often linked to development of emphysema. A less frequent cause is an inherited alpha1-antitryptan deficiency.

24.10 Lung Cancer

Lung cancer is abnormal, uncontrolled cell growth in lung tissues, resulting in a tumor. A tumor in the lung may be primary when it develops in lung tissue. It may be secondary when it spreads (metastasizes) from cancer in other areas of the body such as the liver, brain, or kidneys.

There are two major categories of lung cancer: small cell and non-small cell. Repetitive exposure to inhaled irritants increases a person's risk for lung cancer. Cigarette smoke, occupational exposures, air pollution containing benzopyrenes, and hydrocarbons have all been shown to increase risk.

- **Small Cell:**
  - *Oat Cell:* Fast-growing, early metastasis
- **Non-Small Cell:**
  - *Adenocarcinoma:* Moderate growth rate, early metastasis
  - *Squamous Cell:* Slow-growing, late metastasis
  - *Large Cell:* Fast-growing, early metastasis

24.11 Pleural Effusion

Pleural effusion is the abnormal accumulation of fluid within the pleural space between the parietal and visceral pleura covering the lungs. The fluid may be serous fluid, blood (hemothorax), or pus (empyema). Fluid builds up when the development of the fluid exceeds the body's ability to remove the fluid. Excess fluid inhibits full expansion of the lung.

A large area of fluid buildup will displace the lung tissue, compromising air exchange in the area. As fluid builds up and takes the place of lung tissue, it may push the collapsing lung past the middle (mediastinum) of the chest. This displaces the central structures, compromising the air exchange of the other lung as well.

Causes of pleural effusion are varied and include congestive heart failure, renal failure, malignancy, lupus erythematosus, pulmonary infarction, infection, or trauma. It can also occur as a postoperative complication.

24.12 Pneumonia

Infectious pneumonia may result from a variety of microorganisms and can be community acquired or hospital acquired (nosocomial). A patient can inhale bacteria, viruses, parasites, or irritating agents, or aspirate liquids or foods. He or she can also develop increased mucus production and thickening alveolar fluid as a result of impaired gas exchange. All of these can lead to inflammation of the lower airways.

Organisms commonly associated with infection include *Staphylococcus aureus, Streptococcus pneumoniae, Haemophilus influenza, Mycoplasma pneumoniae, Legionella pneumonia, Chlamydia pneumoniae* (parasite), and *Pseudomonas aeruginosa*.

24.13 Pneumothorax

The pleural sac surrounding the lung normally contains a small amount of fluid to prevent friction as the lungs expand and relax during the respiratory cycle. When air is allowed to enter the pleural space between the lung and the chest wall, a pneumothorax develops. This air pocket takes up space that is normally occupied by lung tissue, causing an area of the lung to partially collapse.

If there is a penetrating chest wound, the patient may have an open pneumothorax, also known as a sucking chest wound (for the sound it makes during breathing).

A closed pneumothorax may be caused by blunt trauma, postcentral line insertion, or postthoracentesis. Spontaneous pneumothorax may be secondary to another disease or occur on its own. As the air accumulates, there may be a partial or complete collapse of the lung—the more air that accumulates, the greater the area of collapse.

If there is a large enough amount of air trapped between the pleural layers, the tension within the area increases. This increase in tension results in pushing the mediastinum toward the unaffected lung, causing it to partially collapse and compromising venous return to the heart. This is a tension pneumothorax.

24.14 Respiratory Acidosis

Hypoventilation, asphyxia, or central nervous system disorders cause a disturbance in the acid-base balance of the patient's blood, resulting in increased carbon dioxide in the blood (hypercapnia). The increase in carbon dioxide in the blood combines with water; this combination releases hydrogen and bicarbonate ions.

The brainstem is stimulated and increases the respiratory drive to blow off carbon dioxide. Over time, the sustained elevated arterial carbon dioxide level causes the kidneys to attempt to compensate by retaining bicarbonate and sodium and excreting hydrogen ions.

24.15 Tuberculosis (TB)

Tuberculosis (TB) is an infectious disease spread by airborne route. Infection is caused by inhalation of droplets that contain the tuberculosis bacteria *(Mycobacterium tuberculosis).*

An infected person can spread the small airborne particles through coughing, sneezing, or talking. Close contact with those affected increases the chances of transmission. Once inhaled, the organism typically settles into the lung, but can infect any organ in the body. The organism has an outer capsule. Primary TB occurs when the patient is initially infected with the mycobacteria. After being inhaled into the lung, the organism causes a localized reaction.

As the macrophages and sensitized T lymphocytes attempt to isolate and kill off the mycobacterium within the lung, damage is also caused to the surrounding lung tissue. A well-defined granulomatous lesion develops that contains the mycobacterium, macrophages, and other cells. Necrotic changes occur within this lesion. Gaseous granulomas develop along lymph node channels during the same time.

These areas create a Ghon's complex, which is a combination of the area initially infected by the airborne bacillus (called the Ghon's focus) and a lymphatic lesion. The majority of people with newly acquired infections and an adequate immune system develop latent infection, as the body walls off the infecting organism within these granulomas. Disease is not active in these patients at this point and will not be transmitted until there is some manifestation of the disease. In patients with inadequate immune response, the TB is progressive, lung tissue destruction continues, and other areas of the lung also become involved. In secondary TB, the disease is reactivated at a later stage.

The patient may be reinfected from droplets or from a prior primary lesion. Since the patient has previously been infected with TB, the immune response is to rapidly wall off the infection. Cavitation of these areas occurs as the organism travels along the airways. Exposure to TB occurs when a person has had recent contact with a person suspected or confirmed of having TB. These patients do not have a positive skin test, signs or symptoms of disease, or chest X-ray changes. They may or may not have disease.

Latent TB infection occurs when a person has a positive tuberculin skin test but no symptoms of disease. Chest X-ray may show granuloma or calcification. TB disease is confirmed when a person has signs and symptoms of TB. The chest X-ray typically has abnormalities in the apical aspects of the lung fields. In HIV patients, other areas may also be affected.

24.16 Acute Respiratory Failure

The lungs are unable to adequately exchange oxygen and carbon dioxide because of insufficient ventilation. The body is not able to maintain enough oxygen or the body may not get rid of enough carbon dioxide. A respiratory illness can deteriorate into acute respiratory failure. Central nervous system depression (because of trauma or medication) or disease can also lead to acute respiratory failure.

24.17 Pulmonary Embolism

Blood flow is obstructed in the lungs caused by a thrombus (blood clot), air, or fat emboli that become stuck in an artery, causing impaired gas exchange. Patients may be predisposed to clot formation, have pooling of blood, or damage to vessel walls, or take certain medications that increase the risk of a thrombus formation. A thrombus is commonly found in vessels in lower extremities.

When a thrombus loosens and travels in the peripheral circulation, it is called an embolus. The embolus travels through the right side of the heart and is sent to the lungs where it lodges in one of the arteries. Depending on the size of the artery that the embolus lodges in, a section of lung will have no blood supply and alveolar function will suffer. As blood supply to an area of the lung diminishes, alveoli collapse, causing atelectasis.

24.18 Influenza

Influenza is a viral infection affecting the respiratory tract that spreads through droplets. The virus can be inhaled or picked up from surfaces through direct contact. Infection can settle into either the upper or lower respiratory tract. The virus causes damage to the upper layers of cells. The natural defenses of the respiratory tract are compromised and it is easier for bacteria to attach to the underlying respiratory tissues.

24.19 Bronchoscopy

Bronchoscopy is used to view the bronchial tree and remove foreign obstructions, obtain tissues for biopsy, or for suctioning fluid. The patient is anesthetized and a bronchoscope is inserted into the patient's mouth and down the trachea and bronchial tree. The bronchoscope contains a tiny video camera and probe that the health care provider manipulates to perform the procedure.

24.20 Pulmonary Angiography

Pulmonary angiography provides a view of the pulmonary circulatory system so that the health care provider can determine the condition of blood flow to the lungs. Radiopaque dye is inserted into the patient's veins after a catheter has been passed through the heart into the pulmonary artery fluoroscopically. The image is watched on a screen as the dye flows through the pulmonary circulatory system.

24.21 Sputum Culture and Sensitivity

Sputum from the patient is cultured to determine which, if any, bacterium is contained in the sputum and determine which antibiotic kills the bacterium. Sputum is collected from the patient in a sterile container and sent to the laboratory, where the sample is smeared in petri dishes and incubated to grow the bacterium. Samples of the bacteria are stained and examined under a microscope to identify the bacterium. The samples are checked periodically, but are usually given 72 hours to complete the testing process. Once identified, bacterium are exposed to known antibiotics to determine which antibiotic kills the bacterium.

24.22 Thoracentesis

Thoracentesis is the removal of fluid from the pleural sac to drain fluid or identify the contents of the fluid. The patient either sits at the edge of the bed or lies on the unaffected side. The affected site is anesthetized. A needle is inserted into the plural sac and fluid is drained using a syringe.

Solved Problems

Respiratory System

24.1 What is acute respiratory distress syndrome (ARDS)?

Patients develop acute respiratory failure. Lungs stiffen as a result of a buildup of fluid in the lungs. Fluid builds up in the tissue of the lungs (interstitium) and the alveoli. This fluid and stiffness impairs the lungs' ability to move air in and out (ventilation). There is an inflammatory response in the tissues of the lungs.

24.2 What causes further impairment to gas exchanges in a patient who has ARDS?

Damage to the surfactant within the alveoli leads to alveolar collapse, further impairing gas exchange.

24.3 What are common causes of ARDS?

This is most commonly caused by shock, sepsis, or as a result of trauma or inhalation injury. Patients may have no history of pulmonary disorders.

24.4 What is asbestosis?

Asbestos fibers enter the lungs, causing inflammation in the bronchioles and the walls of the alveoli. After inhalation, the fibers settle into the lung tissue. Fibrosis develops and ultimately pleural plaques form.

24.5 What is asthma?

The airways become obstructed from either inflammation of the lining of the airways or constriction of the bronchial smooth muscles (bronchospasm).

24.6 What is extrinsic asthma?

Extrinsic asthma, also known as atopic, is caused by allergens such as pollen, animal dander, mold, or dust. It is often accompanied by allergic rhinitis and eczema; this may run in families.

24.7 What is intrinsic asthma?

Intrinsic asthma, also known as nonatopic, is caused by a nonallergic factor such as following a respiratory tract infection, exposure to cold air, changes in air humidity, or respiratory irritants.

24.8 What is atelectasis?

A portion of the lung does not expand completely, decreasing the lung's capacity to exchange gases, which results in decreased oxygenation of blood.

24.9 What are common causes of atelectasis?

Obstruction can be from a mucous plug inside the airway, or a tumor or fluid within the pleural space may be pressing on the airway from the outside. Postoperatively, patients are at risk for atelectasis because of pain, immobility, medications for pain, anesthesia, and lack of deep breathing.

24.10 What is bronchiectasis?

Bronchi and bronchioles become abnormally and permanently dilated, caused by infection and inflammation. This results in excessive production of mucus that obstructs the bronchi. There is some obstruction of the airways and a chronic infection.

24.11 What is bronchitis?

Increased mucus production, caused by infection and airborne irritants that block airways in the lungs, results in the decreased ability to exchange gases.

24.12 What is the difference between acute and chronic bronchitis?

There are two forms of bronchitis: acute bronchitis, in which blockage of the airways is reversible; and chronic bronchitis, in which blockage is not reversible.

24.13 What is cor pulmonale?

In cor pulmonale, the structure and function of the right ventricle are compromised by chronic obstructive pulmonary disease (COPD), obstruction of the airflow into and out of the lungs. The heart tries to compensate, resulting in right-sided heart failure.

24.14 What is the cause of heart failure in cor pulmonale?

The patient has heart failure caused by a primary lung disorder, which causes pulmonary hypertension and enlargement of the right ventricle.

24.15 What symptoms are expected in cor pulmonale?

Patients have symptoms of both the underlying pulmonary disorder and the right-sided heart failure.

24.16 What is chronic obstructive pulmonary disease (COPD)?

COPD consists of chronic bronchitis and emphysema.

24.17 What is emphysema?

Chronic inflammation reduces the flexibility of the walls of the alveoli, resulting in overdistention of the alveolar walls. This causes air to be trapped in the lungs, impeding gas exchange.

24.18 What is a common cause of emphysema?

A common cause of emphysema is smoking.

24.19 What are the two major categories of lung cancer?

Two major categories of lung cancer are small cell and non-small cell.

24.20 What subcategory of lung cancer grows slowly?

Squamous cell is the subcategory of lung cancer that grows slowly.

24.21 What is pleural effusion?

Pleural effusion is abnormal accumulation of fluid within the pleural space between the parietal and visceral pleura covering the lungs.

24.22 What is a result of pleural effusion?

A large area of fluid buildup displaces the lung tissue, compromising air exchange in the area. As fluid builds up and takes the place of lung tissue, it may push the collapsing lung past the middle (mediastinum) of the chest. This displaces the central structures, compromising the air exchange of the other lung as well.

24.23 What are causes of pleural effusion?

Causes of pleural effusion are varied and include congestive heart failure, renal failure, malignancy, lupus erythematosus, pulmonary infarction, infection, or trauma. It can also occur as a postoperative complication.

24.24 What is pneumonia?

Infectious pneumonia may result from a variety of microorganisms and can be community acquired or hospital acquired (nosocomial). A patient can inhale bacteria, viruses, parasites, or irritating agents, or aspirate liquids or foods. He or she can also develop increased mucus production and thickening alveolar fluid as a result of impaired gas exchange. All of these can lead to inflammation of the lower airways.

24.25 What is a pneumothorax?

The pleural sac surrounding the lung normally contains a small amount of fluid to prevent friction as the lungs expand and relax during the respiratory cycle. When air is allowed to enter the pleural space between the lung and the chest wall, a pneumothorax develops

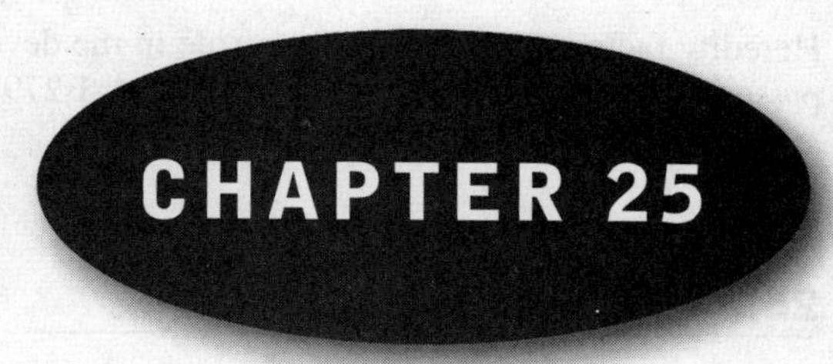

The Immune System

25.1 Definition

Normal functioning of the immune system protects the body against the invasion of outside organisms. A variety of organisms are capable of this; however, not all are harmful. The cells of the immune system recognize organisms that invade the body, then isolate and destroy them.

At times, the immune system is not able to adequately function in this capacity. This results in infection, immunodeficiency disorders, autoimmune disorders, allergies, and hypersensitivity reactions. Lymphocytes are the primary cells of the immune system.

Lymphocytes are divided into B cells and T cells. B cells provide a humoral immune response (antibodies), because they produce an antigen-specific antibody. T cells provide a cellular immune response. Mature T cells are composed of CD4 and CD8 cells. CD8 cells are responsible for destroying foreign and viral inhabited cells, and suppress immunologic functions. CD4 cells, also known as T-helper cells, stimulate immune functions, such as B cells and macrophages. A macrophage is a cell whose functions include ingesting foreign or invading cells.

25.2 Acquired Immunodeficiency Syndrome (AIDS)

The human immunodeficiency virus (HIV) causes malfunction of T cells, which protect the body from invading microorganisms. When it enters a cell, HIV replicates, causing the cell to reproduce more infected cells. It also frequently causes cell death. The CD4 lymphocyte is most often affected, followed by B lymphocytes and macrophages. Immunodeficiency results.

25.3 Anaphylaxis

An allergen, usually food or medication, enters the body causing the release of histamines, resulting in capillaries dilating and smooth muscle contracting. This causes edema, respiratory distress, hypotension, and skin changes, leading to an allergic reaction. Lesser degrees of extreme allergy are urticaria (hives) and angioedema (swelling caused by exudation).

25.4 Ankylosing Spondylitis (AS)

Ankylosing spondylitis (AS) is a progressive form of arthritis that affects <1% of the population. Joints between the spine and pelvis become inflamed, as do some of the ligaments, resulting in instability of the joints.

Heredity factors play an important role in the development of AS. The disease is strongly associated with the presence of histocompatibility antigen HLA-B279 on the chromosomes of affected individuals. It begins in the sacroiliac joints and spreads up the spine.

25.5 Kaposi's Sarcoma

Kaposi's sarcoma (KS) is an overgrowth of blood vessels that leads to malignant tumors and cancer of lymphatic tissue and skin commonly found in patients with AIDS. It is usually seen in cases of advanced AIDS.

25.6 Lymphoma

Functionless and damaged cells of the lymphatic system undergo overgrowth, decreasing the effectiveness of the lymphatic system. The lymphomas are caused by a disruption of cells during differentiation. Diagnosis is made on lymph node biopsy. There are two main types of lymphoma, characterized by painless lymph node swelling:

- **Hodgkin's** Malignant lymphoma characterized by the presence of Reed-Sternberg cells. There are four stages of Hodgkin's disease:
  - *Stage I:* Reed-Sternberg cells appear in one lymph node region.
  - *Stage II:* Reed-Sternberg cells appear in multiple lymph node regions on the same side of the diaphragm.
  - *Stage III:* Reed-Sternberg cells appear in multiple lymph node regions on both sides of the diaphragm.
  - *Stage IV:* Reed-Sternberg cells appear throughout the body.
- **Non-Hodgkin's (NHL)** Cancers of the B lymphocytes that are characterized by the absence of Reed-Sternberg cells.

25.7 Rheumatoid Arthritis

Antibodies from the bloodstream move into the synovial lining of joints, causing joints to swell. The swelling affects the functionality of tendons, bones, and ligaments that move the joint, resulting in pain with movement.

Etiology is unknown, although genetics plays a part. The usual age of onset is 20 to 40 years, and it affects about 2% of the population. Inflammation and nodules around joints are common, usually involving the wrists, hands, knees, and feet.

25.8 Scleroderma

Antibodies attack connective tissues in an autoimmune response. This results in scar tissue (fibrosis) forming on skin, organs, gastrointestinal tract, blood vessels, and muscles, causing systemic sclerosis. It is a chronic disease of unknown etiology, usually seen in 30- to 50-year-old people.

25.9 Mononucleosis

Mononucleosis is a viral syndrome consisting of sore throat, enlarged lymph glands, and fevers. It is usually caused by the Epstein-Barr virus, but sometimes other viruses are the cause such as the cytomegalovirus.

Occasionally, a rash may be seen. The spleen is sometimes enlarged because of sequestration of cells during the immune response.

25.10 Epstein-Barr Virus/Chronic Fatigue Syndrome (CFS)

Chronic fatigue syndrome is a chronic, multisymptom, multisystem syndrome in a previously healthy adult. It results from any of the five known viruses: Epstein-Barr, cytomegalovirus, coxsackievirus B, adenovirus type I, and human herpes virus 6. In an unknown way, the viruses disturb the immune system, which is then unable to adequately fight off the virus.

25.11 Lyme Disease

A bite from a deer tick causes the bacteria (a spirochete) *Borrelia burgdorferi,* to be transmitted into the human bloodstream. The patient presents with fever, myalgias, and the classic bull's-eye rash, erythema chronicum migrans, up to 3 weeks following the bite.

25.12 Septic Shock

Septic shock starts with bacteremia, usually gram-negative bacteria infecting the blood. The sources are usually the genitourinary system, gastrointestinal tract, and lungs. The infection may be underlying for some time before shock develops. Once the cascade from bacteremia to septic shock starts, it may be difficult to halt the process. Shock may occur more quickly in patients who are elderly, immunocompromised, or with other comorbidities. In response to a bacteria infection, TNF-alpha, and other inflammatory chemicals are released into the blood, causing an increase in the blood leaking from vessels into both the infected and uninfected tissues (vascular permeability).

25.13 Systemic Lupus Erythematosus (SLE)

Systemic lupus erythematosus (SLE) is a chronic inflammatory immune disorder affecting the skin and other body organs. Antibodies to DNA and RNA cause an autoimmune inflammatory response, resulting in swelling and pain. It is most common in young women, and has both a strong genetic and gender factor. The etiology is not known.

25.14 Immunologic Blood Studies

The antinuclear antibodies (ANA) test is a screening test for the detection of antibodies to nuclear antigens. Close to 100% of patients with SLE show positive evidence.

- **ESR:** The erythrocyte sedimentation rate is useful in differentiating between inflammatory and neoplastic disease. Serial values are helpful to track disease severity.
- **SS-A and SS-B:** SS-A antibodies can be detected in about 30% of SLE patients. SS-B antibodies have a high specificity for the sicca complex, caused by diminished secretion from glands.
- **Rheumatoid Factor:** Rheumatoid factor is an IgM antibody that is associated with rheumatoid arthritis. Blood is drawn from a vein and a study is conducted to determine if the blood contains this immunoglobulin antibody. Fifty percent of patients with rheumatoid arthritis have this antibody.
- **Scleroderma Autoantibodies:** The scleroderma antibody is found in venous blood of patients who have scleroderma. The autoantibodies are positive in about 25 to 40% of scleroderma patients.

25.15 Lymphangiography

This test produces a radiographic image of the lymphatic system to determine if there are any abnormalities such as edema of the legs, Hodgkin's and non-Hodgkin's lymphoma, lymphadenopathy, and lymphatic metastases. The results are useful in the staging of lymphoma and Hodgkin's lymphoma and to determine the efficacy of treatment.

Solved Problems

Immune System

25.1 What are B cells?

B cells provide a humoral immune response, because they produce an antigen-specific antibody.

25.2 What are T cells?

T cells provide a cellular immune response.

25.3 What are CD8 cells?

CD8 cells are responsible for destroying foreign and viral inhabited cells, and suppressing immunologic functions.

25.4 What are CD4 cells?

CD4 cells, also known as T-helper cells, stimulate immune functions, such as B cells and macrophages.

25.5 What is a macrophage?

A macrophage is a cell whose functions include ingesting foreign or invading cells.

25.6 What is acquired immunodeficiency syndrome (AIDS)?

AIDS is a disease caused when the human immunodeficiency virus (HIV) enters a cell, and HIV replicates, causing the cell to reproduce more infected cells. It also frequently causes cell death.

25.7 What is a major result of the human immunodeficiency virus (HIV)?

HIV causes malfunction of T cells, which protect the body from invading microorganisms. The CD4 lymphocyte is most often affected, followed by B lymphocytes and macrophages. Immunodeficiency results.

25.8 What is anaphylaxis?

An allergen, usually food or medication, enters the body, causing the release of histamines, which result in capillaries dilating and smooth muscle contracting. This results in edema, respiratory distress, hypotension, and skin changes, leading to an allergic reaction. Lesser degrees of extreme allergy are urticaria (hives) and angioedema (swelling caused by exudation).

25.9 What is ankylosing spondylitis (AS)?

AS is a progressive form of arthritis that affects $<1\%$ of the population. Joints between the spine and pelvis become inflamed, as do some of the ligaments, resulting in instability of the joints.

25.10 What is a Kaposi's sarcoma (KS)?

KS is an overgrowth of blood vessels that leads to malignant tumors and cancer of lymphatic tissue and skin commonly found in patients with AIDS. It is usually seen in cases of advanced AIDS.

25.11 What is lymphoma?

Functionless and damaged cells of the lymphatic system undergo overgrowth, decreasing the effectiveness of the lymphatic system.

25.12 What is a common sign of lymphoma?

Painless lymph node swelling is a common sign of lymphoma.

25.13 What are the two main types of lymphoma?

Two main types of lymphoma are Hodgkin's and non-Hodgkin's lymphoma.

25.14 What is Hodgkin's lymphoma?

Hodgkin's lymphoma is malignant lymphoma characterized by the presence of Reed-Sternberg cells.

25.15 What is non-Hodgkin's lymphoma (NHL)?

NHL is cancer of the B lymphocytes and is characterized by the absence of Reed-Sternberg cells.

25.16 What is rheumatoid arthritis?

Antibodies from the bloodstream move into the synovial lining of joints, causing joints to swell. The swelling affects the functionality of tendons, bones, and ligaments that move the joint, resulting in pain with movement.

25.17 What is scleroderma?

Antibodies attack connective tissues in an autoimmune response. This results in scar tissue (fibrosis) forming on skin, organs, gastrointestinal tract, blood vessels, and muscles, causing systemic sclerosis.

25.18 What is mononucleosis?

Mononucleosis is a viral syndrome consisting of sore throat, enlarged lymph glands, and fevers.

25.19 What is chronic fatigue syndrome (CFS)?

CFS is a chronic, multisymptom, multisystem syndrome in a previously healthy adult. It results from any of the five known viruses: Epstein-Barr, cytomegalovirus, coxsackievirus B, adenovirus type I, and human herpes virus 6. In an unknown way, the viruses disturb the immune system, which is then unable to adequately fight off the virus.

25.20 What is Lyme disease?

A bite from a deer tick causes the bacteria (a spirochete) *Borrelia burgdorferi,* to be transmitted into the human bloodstream. This is referred to as Lyme disease. The patient presents with fever, myalgias and the classic bull's-eye rash, erythema chronicum migrans up to 3 weeks following the bite.

25.21 What is septic shock?

Septic shock starts with bacteremia, usually gram-negative bacteria infecting the blood. The sources are usually the genitourinary system, gastrointestinal tract, and lungs. The infection may be underlying for some time before shock develops. Once the cascade from bacteremia to septic shock starts, it may be difficult to halt the process.

25.22 What is systemic lupus erythematosus (SLE)?

SLE is a chronic inflammatory immune disorder affecting the skin and other body organs. Antibodies to DNA and RNA cause an autoimmune inflammatory response, resulting in swelling and pain.

25.23 What is the usefulness of knowing the erythrocyte sedimentation rate (ESR)?

The ESR is useful in differentiating between inflammatory and neoplastic disease.

25.24 What is the rheumatoid factor?

The rheumatoid factor is an IgM antibody that is associated with rheumatoid arthritis. Fifty percent of the patients with rheumatoid arthritis have this antibody.

25.25 What is lymphangiography?

This test produces a radiographic image of the lymphatic system to determine if there are any abnormalities, such as edema of the legs, Hodgkin's lymphoma, non-Hodgking lymphoma, lymphadenopathy, and lymphatic metastases.

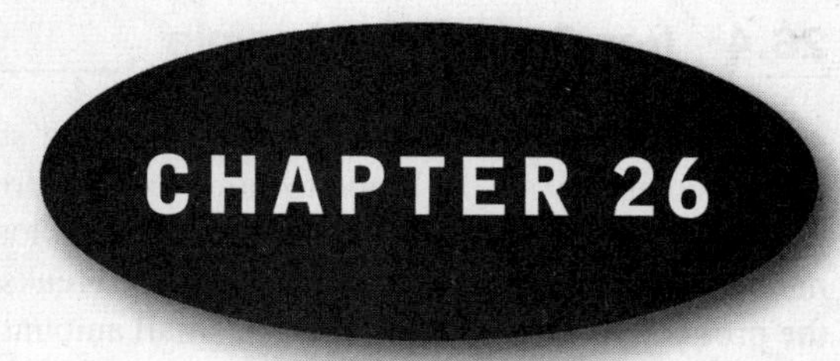

The Hematologic System

26.1 Definition

The hematologic system refers to the blood and blood-forming organs. The formation of red blood cells (RBCs), white blood cells (WBCs), and platelets begins in the bone marrow. Stem cells are produced in the bone marrow. Initially, these cells are not differentiated and may become RBCs, WBCs, or platelets. In the next stage of development, the stem cell becomes committed to a particular precursor cell, to become either a myeloid or lymphoid type of cell, and differentiates into a particular cell type when in the presence of a specific growth factor.

The spleen is found in the left upper quadrant of the abdomen. The spleen filters whole blood. It removes old and imperfect WBCs, lymphocytes and macrophages, and RBCs. The spleen also breaks down hemoglobin and stores of RBCs and platelets.

The liver is found in the right upper quadrant of the abdomen and is the main production site for many of the clotting factors, including prothrombin. Normal liver function is important for vitamin K production in the intestinal tract. Vitamin K is necessary for clotting factors VII, IX, X, and prothrombin.

26.2 Anemia

A low hemoglobin or RBC count results in decreased oxygen-carrying capability of the blood. This may be because of blood loss, damage to the RBCs due to altered hemoglobin or destruction (hemolysis), nutritional deficiency (iron, vitamin B_{12}, folic acid), lack of RBC production, or bone marrow failure. Some patients have a family history of anemia caused by genetic transmission, such as thalassemia or sickle cell.

26.3 Aplastic Anemia (Pancytopenia)

The bone marrow stops producing a sufficient amount of RBCs, WBCs, and platelets, thereby increasing the risk of infection and hemorrhage. The red cells remaining in circulation are normal in size and color. This may be because of chemical exposure, high-dose radiation exposure, or exposure to toxins. Cancer treatments such as radiation therapy and chemotherapeutic agents may suppress bone marrow function, which results in anemia (low RBC), thrombocytopenia (low platelets), and leukopenia (low WBC). The cause may also be unknown or idiopathic.

26.4 Iron Deficiency Anemia

A lower-than-normal amount of iron in blood serum results in decreased formation of hemoglobin and a decreased ability for the blood to carry oxygen. Iron stores are typically depleted first, followed by serum iron levels. Iron deficiency may be a result of blood loss, dietary deficiency, or increased demand because of pregnancy or lactation. As RBCs age, the body breaks them down and the iron is released. This iron is reused for the production of new blood cells. A small amount of iron is lost daily through the gastrointestinal tract, necessitating dietary replacement. When RBCs are produced without a sufficient amount of iron, the cells are smaller and paler than usual.

26.5 Pernicious Anemia

The body is unable to absorb vitamin B_{12}, which is needed to make RBCs, resulting in a decreased RBC count. More common in people of northern European descent, the anemia typically develops in adulthood. The intrinsic factor is normally secreted by the parietal cells of the gastric mucosa and is necessary to allow intestinal absorption of vitamin B_{12}. Destruction of the gastric mucosa because of an autoimmune response results in loss of parietal cells within the stomach. The ability of vitamin B_{12} to bind with intrinsic factor is lost, decreasing the amount that is absorbed. Typical onset is between the ages of 40 and 60.

26.6 Disseminated Intravascular Coagulation (DIC)

Blood coagulates through the entire body within the vascular compartment. This depletes platelets and the body's ability to coagulate, resulting in an increased risk of hemorrhage. It occurs as a complication of some other condition. The coagulation sequence is activated, causing many microthrombi to develop throughout the body. The clots that form are the result of coagulation proteins and platelets, resulting in the risk of bleeding or severe hemorrhage. It is often caused by obstetric complications, post trauma, sepsis, cancer, or shock.

26.7 Hemophilia

The patient is missing a coagulation factor that is essential for normal blood clotting and as a result, the blood does not clot when the patient bleeds. It is an X-linked recessive inherited disorder, passed on so that it presents symptoms in males, and rarely in females. Hemophilia A is the result of missing clotting factor VIII. Hemophilia B is the result of missing clotting factor IX and is also known as Christmas disease.

26.8 Leukemia

Replacement of bone marrow by abnormal cells results in unregulated proliferation of immature WBCs entering the circulatory system. These leukemic cells may also enter the liver, spleen, or lymph nodes, causing these areas to enlarge.

Leukemia is classified according to the type of cell from which it is derived, lymphocytic or myelocytic, and as either acute or chronic. Lymphocytic leukemias involve immature lymphocytes originating in the bone marrow and typically infiltrate the spleen, lymph nodes, or central nervous system. Myelogenous or myelocytic leukemia involves the myeloid stem cells in the bone marrow and interferes with the maturation of all blood cell types (granulocytes, erythrocytes, thrombocytes).

The exact cause of leukemia is unknown. There is a higher incidence in people who have been exposed to high levels of radiation, have had exposure to benzene, or have a history of aggressive chemotherapy for a different type of cancer. There may be a genetic predisposition to develop acute leukemia. Patients with

Down's syndrome, Fanconi's anemia, or a family history of leukemia also have a higher-than-average incidence of this disease.

26.9 Multiple Myeloma

A malignancy of the plasma cells causes an excessive amount of plasma cells in the bone marrow. Masses within the bone marrow cause destructive lesions in the bone. Normal bone marrow function is reduced as the abnormal plasma cells continue to grow. Immune function is diminished and the patient develops anemia. The disease typically affects older adults.

26.10 Polycythemia Vera

Polycythemia vera is a myeloproliferative disorder that results in an overproduction of blood cells and a thickening of blood. The hallmarks of polycythemia vera include excessive production of RBCs, WBCs, and platelets. The excess of cells present in the blood causes problems with the flow of blood through vessels, especially the smaller ones. There is an increase in peripheral vascular resistance causing increased pressure, and vascular stasis in the smaller vessels, potentially causing thrombosis or tissue hypoxia. Organ damage may result because of these changes.

26.11 Sickle Cell Anemia

This is an autosomal recessive disorder in which an abnormal gene causes damage to the RBC membrane. The abnormal hemoglobin within the RBC is called hemoglobin S. Dehydration or drying of the RBC makes it more vulnerable to sickling (forming a crescent-like shape), as do hypoxemia and acidosis. Hemolytic anemia results as RBCs are destroyed because of the damage to the outer membrane. The sickled cells can also clump together, causing difficulty getting through the smaller vessels.

26.12 Deep Vein Thrombosis (DVT)

Thrombophlebitis, or the formation of a clot within the vein, commonly occurs within the deep veins in the legs, and may also occur in the arms. Initially platelets and white cells clump together, sticking to the inside of the vessel wall. As blood flows over the area, other cells may deposit on the area, making the thrombus larger. Compression of blood flow that increases the venous pressure or sluggishness of the blood flow can increase the risk of clot formation. Immobility, obesity, or hormonal changes such as pregnancy can all contribute to increased risk.

26.13 Idiopathic Thrombocytopenic Purpura (ITP)

Idiopathic thrombocytopenic purpura (ITP) is an autoimmune disorder in which antibodies are developed in the patient's own platelets. Antibodies attach to the platelets and macrophages within the spleen. The body destroys the platelets within the spleen. ITP is typically more common in women and becomes chronic in adults who are in early to mid-adulthood.

26.14 Bone Marrow Biopsy

Bone marrow biopsy is the removal of bone marrow by needle or aspiration to determine blood cell formation.

Solved Problems

Hematologic System

26.1 What are stem cells?

Stem cells are produced in the bone marrow. Initially, these cells are not differentiated and may become RBCs, WBCs, or platelets. In the next stage of development, the stem cell becomes committed to a particular precursor cell, to become either a myeloid or lymphoid type of cell and will differentiate into a particular cell type when in the presence of a specific growth factor.

26.2 What is the function of the spleen?

The spleen filters whole blood. It removes old and imperfect WBCs, lymphocytes and macrophages, and RBCs. The spleen also breaks down hemoglobin and stores of RBCs and platelets.

26.3 What is anemia?

A low hemoglobin or RBC count results in decreased oxygen carrying capability of the blood.

26.4 What causes anemia?

This may be caused by blood loss, damage to RBCs resulting from altered hemoglobin or destruction (hemolysis), nutritional deficiency (iron, vitamin B_{12}, folic acid), lack of RBC production, or bone marrow failure. Some patients have a family history of anemia caused by genetic transmission.

26.5 What is aplastic anemia?

The bone marrow stops producing a sufficient amount of RBCs, WBCs, and platelets, thereby increasing the risk of infection and hemorrhage.

26.6 What is a common cause of aplastic anemia?

Cancer treatments are a common cause of aplastic anemia.

26.7 What is iron deficiency anemia?

A lower-than-normal amount of iron in blood serum results in decreased formation of hemoglobin and a decreased ability for the blood to carry oxygen. Iron stores are typically depleted first, followed by serum iron levels.

26.8 What causes iron deficiency?

Iron deficiency may be caused by blood loss, dietary deficiency, or increased demand because of pregnancy or lactation.

26.9 Where does the body get a large amount of iron?

As RBCs age, the body breaks them down and the iron is released. This iron is reused for the production of new blood cells. A small amount of iron is lost daily through the gastrointestinal tract, necessitating dietary replacement.

26.10 What is a pernicious anemia?

The body is unable to absorb vitamin B_{12}, which is needed to make RBCs, resulting in a decreased RBC count.

26.11 What enables the body to absorb vitamin B_{12}?

The intrinsic factor is normally secreted by the parietal cells of the gastric mucosa and is necessary to allow intestinal absorption of vitamin B_{12}.

26.12 What is a common cause of pernicious anemia?

Destruction of the gastric mucosa because of an autoimmune response results in loss of parietal cells within the stomach.

26.13 What is disseminated intravascular coagulation (DIC)?

Blood coagulates through the entire body within the vascular compartment. This depletes platelets and the body's ability to coagulate, resulting in an increased risk of hemorrhage.

26.14 What is the cause of disseminated intravascular coagulation?

DIC is often caused by obstetric complications, post trauma, sepsis, cancer, or shock.

26.15 What is hemophilia?

The patient is missing a coagulation factor that is essential for normal blood clotting and as a result, the blood does not clot when the patient bleeds.

26.16 What is leukemia?

Replacement of bone marrow by abnormal cells results in unregulated proliferation of immature WBCs entering the circulatory system. These leukemic cells may also enter the liver, spleen, or lymph nodes, causing these areas to enlarge.

26.17 What is myelocytic leukemia?

Myelogenous or myelocytic leukemia involves the myeloid stem cells in the bone marrow and interferes with the maturation of all blood cell types.

26.18 What are lymphocytic leukemias?

Lymphocytic leukemias involve immature lymphocytes originating in the bone marrow and typically infiltrate the spleen, lymph nodes, or central nervous system.

26.19 How is leukemia classified?

Leukemia is classified according to the type of cell it is derived from, lymphocytic or myelocytic, and as either acute or chronic.

26.20 What is the exact cause of leukemia?

The exact cause of leukemia is unknown.

26.21 What is multiple myeloma?

A malignancy of the plasma cells causes an excessive amount of plasma cells in the bone marrow. Masses within the bone marrow cause destructive lesions in the bone. Normal bone marrow function is reduced as the abnormal plasma cells continue to grow. Immune function is diminished and the patient develops anemia.

26.22 What is polycythemia vera?

Polycythemia vera is a myeloproliferative disorder that results in an overproduction of blood cells and a thickening of blood. The hallmarks of polycythemia vera include excessive production of RBCs, WBCs, and platelets. The excess of cells present in the blood causes problems with the flow of blood through vessels, especially the smaller ones.

26.23 What is sickle cell anemia?

Sickle cell anemia is an autosomal recessive disorder in which an abnormal gene causes damage to the RBC membrane. The abnormal hemoglobin within the RBC is called hemoglobin S. Dehydration or drying of the RBC makes it more vulnerable to sickling (forming a crescent-like shape), as do hypoxemia and acidosis. Hemolytic anemia results as RBCs are destroyed because of the damage to the outer membrane. The sickled cells can also clump together, causing difficulty getting through the smaller vessels.

26.24 What is deep vein thrombosis (DVT)?

Thrombophlebitis, or the formation of a clot within the vein, commonly occurs within the deep veins in the legs, and may also occur in the arms. Initially platelets and white cells clump together, sticking to the inside of the vessel wall. As blood flows over the area, other cells may deposit onto the area, making the thrombus larger. Compression of blood flow that increases the venous pressure or sluggishness of the blood flow can increase the risk of clot formation.

26.25 What is idiopathic thrombocytopenic purpura (ITP)?

ITP is an autoimmune disorder in which antibodies are developed to the patient's own platelets. Antibodies attach to the platelets and macrophages within the spleen. The body destroys the platelets within the spleen.

The Nervous System

27.1 Definition

The nervous system is divided into the central and peripheral nervous systems. The central nervous system (CNS) is composed of the brain and spinal cord. The peripheral nervous system (PNS) contains the spinal nerves and peripheral nerves. The basic component of the nervous system is the nerve cell or neuron.

A neuron is composed of the nucleus within the cell body, a dendrite (that receives the signal), an axon (the extension of the cell that can pass on an impulse to the next nerve cell), and the axon terminals (that can transmit the signals to other cells). The messages are sent from one nerve cell to another, crossing a synapse (or gap) between cells.

Neurotransmitters are chemicals released by the presynaptic neuron to enhance the communication between nerve cells. There are specific receptor sites for the different neurotransmitters on the postsynaptic neuron. Electrically charged ions transmit signals along the cell membranes of the nerve cells. A myelin coating on the outer surface of the nerve cells helps to speed the transmission along the nerve cells. This myelin coating also gives a white color to the nerve cells.

Some neurons are afferent neurons. They carry sensory information from the peripheral areas of the body to the CNS. These neurons do not have dendrites. Motor neurons that transmit information from the CNS to the muscles or glands are efferent neurons.

The brain is protected within the skull. The outermost layer of the brain is the cerebral cortex, made up primarily of neural cell bodies, giving a gray appearance. The cerebral cortex is divided into right and left hemispheres and into frontal, parietal, occipital, and temporal lobes. The frontal lobe has motor and premotor areas, as well as Broca's area, which controls speech articulation, behavior, moral decision making, and emotional outbursts. The parietal area interprets sensory stimuli, pain, and touch. The temporal lobe is where language is interpreted (Wernicke's area). It also processes auditory information, and controls memory formation and storage.

The occipital lobe houses the visual cortex. The diencephalon includes the thalamus, hypothalamus, and basal ganglia. The thalamus relays the sensory information from the body to the appropriate part of the cerebral cortex. Descending messages from the cerebral cortex are passed through the thalamus to the body.

The hypothalamus controls neuroendocrine function and maintains homeostasis, or constancy, within the body. The basal ganglia control highly skilled movements that require precision without intentional thought. The brain stem is comprised of the pons, medulla oblongata, and midbrain. The spinal column is protected within the vertebral column. Both motor and sensory fibers are found within the spinal column. Motor nerves are located along the anterior horns and sensory nerves are located along the posterior horns of the spinal column. The motor nerve fibers are more protected from traumatic injury this way.

If a patient sustains an external injury to the back that damages the spinal column, the first area to be impacted will be the sensory nerves, hopefully maintaining motor function. If enough damage has occurred, then both sensory and motor function will be lost. Peripheral nerve fibers leave the spinal column to travel to the rest of the body. Impulses travel from the CNS to muscle fibers to control voluntary motion and involuntary function of organs. Impulses are also sent from the body to the CNS for input.

27.2 Head Injury

The patient experiences a trauma to the head. The resulting injury may be a minor scalp laceration or a major internal injury with or without a skull fracture. There may be internal hemorrhage or cerebral edema, resulting in hypoxia and a decrease in cognitive and functional capabilities.

There are a variety of injuries that may be sustained. Open head injuries are typical of projectile wounds from gunshots or knives. Closed head injuries are typical of trauma from falls, motor vehicle accidents, sports, or fights.

Concussion involves a blow to the head in which there is a bruising-type injury as the brain is thrust against the inside of the skull. The point of injury where the brain makes impact against the skull is referred to as a coup injury.

There is also a contrecoup injury that occurs on the side opposite of the area that was impacted as the head recoils away from the point of impact and the brain is thrust against the inside of the skull at the opposite point of the head, resulting in injury there as well.

Patients with concussion may experience a transient loss of consciousness associated with bradycardia, or slowing of the heart rate; low blood pressure; slow, shallow breathing; amnesia of the injury and the events immediately following the injury; headache; and temporary loss of mental focus.

Cerebral contusion is a more serious injury than concussion. Greater damage is done to the brain, cerebral edema or hemorrhage may occur and lead to necrosis. Patients typically have longer loss of consciousness with a cerebral contusion. Hemorrhages can occur at a variety of levels: between the skull and the outer coverings (dura) of the brain, within the layers covering the brain, or within the brain tissue. The bleeding may occur acutely, at the time of injury, or hours to weeks later.

An epidural hematoma happens at the time of injury from an arterial site. The blood accumulates between the skull and the dura mater, or the outermost layer covering the brain. The site is often in the temporal area. The patient is typically awake and talking immediately after the blow to the head. Within a short time, the patient becomes unstable and then unconscious.

Emergency neurosurgery is necessary to relieve the pressure and stop the bleeding. Subdural hematoma is typically bleeding from a venous source into the area below the dura mater and above the arachnoid mater. This may occur acutely in some patients, but can also occur as a slow, chronic bleed, especially in the elderly patient. The elderly patient with a chronic bleed may have a significant amount of blood accumulate before symptoms occur because of age-related changes in the volume of brain tissue.

A subarachnoid hemorrhage causes blood to accumulate within the area below the arachnoid mater and above the pia mater. The cerebrospinal fluid is found in this area. An intracerebral bleed is an accumulation of blood within the tissues of the brain. This may be the result of a shearing force on the brain tissue from a twisting motion between the upper part of the brain (cerebrum) and the brainstem or tearing of small vessels within the brain. There will be associated edema and elevation of intracranial pressure.

Simple skull fractures are displaced and do not require specific intervention. Depressed skull fractures have bone fragments that have been broken off from the skull and pressed down toward the brain tissue. These fractures need to be corrected surgically. A basilar skull fracture has classic signs that include periorbital bruising (raccoon sign), blood behind the ear drum (Battle's sign), and leaking of cerebrospinal fluid from the nose or ear (check for glucose content to distinguish from a runny nose).

27.3 Amyotrophic Lateral Sclerosis (ALS)

Amyotrophic lateral sclerosis (ALS) is commonly called Lou Gehrig's disease and is a progressive, degenerative disorder that involves both the upper and lower motor neurons. There is no change in mental status or sensory function with the disease, although the disease does result in paralysis of the motor system, except the eyes. As the disease progresses, families often can communicate with the patient through eye movements. Males are affected more commonly than females. The disorder may present at any age, but onset is usually between age 40 and the late sixties. There is a familial form of the disease that has been linked to an abnormality in chromosome 21.

27.4 Bell's Palsy

This is an acute idiopathic facial paralysis of the seventh cranial nerve that affects one side of the face. Often caused by inflammation, the disorder is more common in diabetic patients. One side of the face is paralyzed, making the patient unable to close the eyelid, raise the eyebrow, or smile on the affected side of the face. Some patients experience pain around the ear on the affected side. The patient may have an associated change in taste.

27.5 Brain Abscess

Collection of pus creates a space-occupying area within the brain. Symptoms are similar to any other space-occupying lesion. The infection may be a primary site within the brain or may have traveled from nearby sites such as the ear or sinuses through bone erosion. It may also enter the brain via the systemic circulation from any infected site in the body, such as the lungs in bronchiectasis.

The organism causes a local inflammatory reaction; there is pus and liquefaction of the affected tissue. Cerebral edema of the surrounding tissue occurs. The area becomes encapsulated within 10 to 14 days from the onset of the infection. Infections are typically streptococci, staphylococci, anaerobes, or mixed organism. Immunocompromised patients may have fungal or yeast present in the abscess. Up to 20% of patients may have more than one abscess.

27.6 Brain Tumor

A brain tumor is a growth of abnormal cells within the brain tissue. The tumor may be a primary site that originated in the brain or a secondary site that has metastasized from a cancer site elsewhere in the body. Because the tumor is growing within the confined space of the skull, the patient eventually develops signs of increased intracranial pressure. Some cell types grow faster than others; patients with more aggressive, fast-growing cancers develop symptoms more quickly.

27.7 Cerebral Aneurysm

A cerebral aneurysm is a balloon-like outpouching caused by a congenital or developed weakness in a cerebral artery. Trauma, infection, or vessel wall lesions caused by atherosclerosis can all lead to the development of an aneurysm. Increased pressure within the vessel lumen may cause the aneurysm to rupture, causing significant intracranial bleeding.

27.8 Encephalitis

Encephalitis is an inflammation of the brain tissue, most often caused by a virus, although it can also result from bacteria, fungus, or protozoa. In the case of viral encephalitis, the patient typically had viral symptoms before the current illness. The virus enters the CNS via the bloodstream and begins to reproduce. Inflammation in the area follows, causing damage to the neurons.

Demyelination of the nerve fibers in the affected area and hemorrhage, edema, and necrosis occur, which create small cavities within the brain tissue. Herpes simplex virus 1, cytomegalovirus, echovirus, coxsackievirus, and herpes zoster can all cause encephalitis. Some forms of encephalitis can be transmitted by insects such as mosquitoes or ticks to humans, and can cause diseases such as West Nile virus, St. Louis encephalitis, or equine encephalitis.

27.9 Guillain-Barré Syndrome

Guillain-Barré syndrome is an acute, progressive autoimmune condition that affects the peripheral nerves. Symptoms occur as the myelin surrounding the axon on the peripheral nerves is damaged from the autoimmune effect. The disease typically follows a viral infection, surgery, other acute illness, or immunization by a couple of weeks.

Ascending Guillain-Barré exhibits muscle weakness and/or paralysis begins in the distal lower extremities and travels upward. Patient may also experience altered sensory perception in the same areas, such as the sensation of crawling, tingling, burning, or pain. The progression of symptoms may take hours or days.

Descending Guillain-Barré begins with muscles in the face, jaw, or throat and travels downward. Respiratory compromise is a concern as the paralysis reaches the level of the intercostal muscles and diaphragm. Breathing can become compromised more quickly in patients with descending disease. Level of consciousness, mental status, personality, and pupil size are not affected.

27.10 Huntington's Disease (Chorea)

Huntington's disease is a degenerative disease that presents with a gradual onset of involuntary, jerking movements (chorea) and a progressive decline in mental ability, resulting in behavioral changes and dementia. The disease is transmitted genetically, as an autosomal dominant trait located on chromosome 4. Family members of patients can have genetic testing done to identify the presence of the gene. The symptoms typically appear between the ages of 30 and 50 years.

27.11 Meningitis

Meningitis is the inflammation of the meningeal coverings of the brain and spinal cord, most commonly caused by bacteria or viral origin, although it can also be caused by fungus, protozoa, or toxic exposure. Bacterial meningitis is the most common and is typically a result of *Streptococcus pneumoniae* (pneumococcal), *Neisseria meningitides* (meningococcal), or *Haemophilus influenzae*.

The incidence of *H. influenzae* meningitis infections has decreased since the vaccine against *H. influenzae* began to be used routinely in infants in the early 1990s. Other organisms that can cause bacterial meningitis include *Staphylococcus aureus, Escherichia coli,* and *Pseudomonas*.

Organisms typically travel either through the bloodstream to the CNS or enter by direct contamination (skull fracture or extension from sinus infections). Bacterial meningitis is more common in colder months when upper respiratory tract infections are more common.

People in close living conditions, such as prisons, military barracks, or college dorms are at greater risk for outbreaks of bacterial meningitis due to the likelihood of transmission. Viral meningitis may follow other viral infections, such as mumps, herpes simplex or zoster, enterovirus, and measles.

Viral meningitis is often a self-limiting illness. Patients who are immunocompromised have an increased risk for contracting fungal meningitis. This may travel from the bloodstream to the CNS or by direct contamination. *Cryptococcus neoformans* may be the causative organism in these patients.

27.12 Multiple Sclerosis (MS)

Multiple sclerosis (MS) is an autoimmune disease that results in demyelination of the white matter of the nervous system. Nerve impulses travel along the myelin coating on the outside of the nerve cells. With the disruption in the myelin on the outside of the nerve cells, the transmission of information from cell to cell within the nervous system is altered.

The patient's sensations, movements, or mental function may be affected. A patient with relapsing-remitting disease will have episodes of exacerbation when symptoms occur and then months or years of symptom-free episodes.

A portion of these patients progress to enter a disease state that has a steady pattern of deterioration without relation to periodic exacerbations; this is referred to as secondary progressive disease. Other patients have primary progressive disease and develop steady deterioration from the onset of the disease.

27.13 Myasthenia Gravis

Myasthenia gravis is a disorder of the PNS involving antibodies that have been produced by the body; they bind to receptor sites that normally bind acetylcholine. This prevents the acetylcholine from binding to the receptor sites on the skeletal muscle, causing abnormal muscle contraction in the affected area.

The areas of the body most commonly affected by the autoimmune disease include the muscles in the eyes, face, lips, tongue, throat, and neck, resulting in weakness and fatigue of these areas. The disease does not seem to be hereditary, but does have a family tendency toward autoimmune disorders.

The majority of patients have a hyperplasia (excessive growth of normal cells) of the thymus gland. Myasthenia gravis is more likely to develop in young adults and is more common in women.

27.14 Parkinson's Disease

There is a gradual degeneration of the midbrain area known as the substantia nigra. The neurons use the neurotransmitter dopamine to send their signals from cell to cell. The loss of neurons within the substantia nigra continues and results in diminished voluntary fine motor skills owing to dopamine loss. There is also development of sympathetic noradrenergic lesions, causing norepinephrine loss within the sympathetic nervous system.

There is excess effect of the excitatory neurotransmitter acetylcholine on the neurons; this causes increased muscle tone, leading to rigidity and tremors. There seems to be a genetic tendency toward development of Parkinson's disease. Environmental factors such as exposure to airborne contaminants, occupational chemicals, toxins, or a virus have been implicated in the development of the disease. The typical age of onset is after the fifth decade of life.

27.15 Spinal Cord Injury

Injury to the spinal cord results in compression, twisting, severing, or pulling on the spinal cord. The damage to the cord may involve the entire thickness of the cord (complete), or only a partial area of the spinal cord (incomplete). The most common cause of spinal cord injury is trauma.

Any level of the spinal cord may have been affected by the injury. Loss of sensation, motor control, or reflexes may occur below the level of injury or within one to two vertebrae or spinal nerves above the level of injury. The loss may be unilateral or bilateral. Damage to the vertebrae may have occurred at the same time as the spinal cord injury.

Swelling because of the initial trauma may make the injury seem more severe than it actually is. When the initial swelling resolves, the actual degree of permanent injury can be more accurately assessed.

27.16 Stroke

A stroke is also known as a cerebrovascular accident (CVA) or a brain attack. Blood supply is interrupted to part of the brain, causing brain cells to die. This results in the patient losing brain function in the affected area.

Interruption is usually caused by an obstruction of arterial blood flow (ischemic stroke), such as formation of a blood clot, but can also be caused by a leaking or ruptured blood vessel (hemorrhagic stroke). A blood clot may develop from a piece of unstable plaque lining a vessel wall that breaks free, or an embolus that travels from elsewhere in the body and lodges within the vessel.

The bleeding may occur as a result of trauma or spontaneously, as in the setting of uncontrolled hypertension. Ischemia occurs when insufficient blood is getting to the brain tissue. This leads to lack of available oxygen (hypoxia) and glucose (hypoglycemia) for the brain. When these nutrients are not available for a sustained period, the brain cells die, causing an area of infarction.

Permanent deficits result from infarction. There is increased risk for stroke in patients with a history of hypertension, diabetes mellitus, high cholesterol, atrial fibrillation, obesity, smoking, or oral contraceptive use. Patients may also experience a transient ischemic attack (TIA) in which the symptoms result from a temporary problem with blood flow to a specific area of the brain. The symptoms have a duration between a few minutes and 24 hours.

27.17 Seizure Disorder

This is a disorder that involves a sudden episode of abnormal, uncontrolled discharge of the electrical activity of the neurons within the brain. The patient may experience a variety of symptoms depending on the type of seizure and the cause.

Seizures may be a symptom of another condition—such as a tumor or stroke that has increased the intracranial pressure, a metabolic disorder, withdrawal from alcohol or drugs—or may result from a chronic seizure disorder such as epilepsy.

Before the seizure, the patient may experience an aura, a sensory alteration involving sight, sound, or smell. After the seizure, the patient enters a postictal stage in which there may be confusion and the patient is often fatigued. The patient may not recall any of the seizure or the time immediately surrounding the seizure.

27.18 Computed Tomography (CT) With or Without Contrast

The practitioner may do an initial test without contrast for first images and then give contrast and repeat images to compare. This is done to check for bleeding, tumor, abscess, infarction, and hydrocephalus.

27.19 Computed Tomography Angiography (CTA)

Computed tomography angiography (CTA) creates a three-dimensional reconstruction of the vasculature within the area imaged.

27.20 Cerebral Angiography

Contrast material is injected to visualize the cerebral circulation, carotid, and vertebral arteries. This test is done to identify aneurysms, arteriovenous malformations, traumatic injuries, strictures, occlusions, and tumors. The head is immobilized during the test.

Wire is inserted via the femoral arterial site and passed to the carotid or vertebral vessel under fluoroscopic guidance. Contrast dye is injected so that three-dimensional images can be obtained. After the test, the practitioner needs to monitor vital signs and perform neurologic checks and neurovascular checks of the extremity (capillary refill, peripheral pulses, skin color, and temperature). The practitioner must also check for bleeding at the site.

27.21 Electroencephalography (EEG)

The EEG records the electrical activity from the cerebral hemispheres of the brain and creates a graphic recording. It determines general brain activity as well as the site of origin of seizure activity. It is also used to diagnose sleep disorders and determine brain death.

27.22 Lumbar Puncture

A spinal needle is inserted into the subarachnoid space at levels of L3–L4 or L4–L5 with the patient lying on the side with knees drawn up to his or her chest. This test is performed under local anesthesia. It is done to obtain pressure readings, obtain cerebrospinal fluid for analysis, inject contrast material or air for diagnostic tests, inject medications, or reduce increased intracranial pressure. The patient must lie flat for several hours after the procedure to reduce the risk of spinal headache caused by leakage of spinal fluid. The practitioner should encourage oral fluid intake.

27.23 Magnetic Resonance Imaging (MRI) With Gadolinium

The MRI is done to detect differences in tissue integrity, tumors, and disk disease. Because of the use of a magnetic field to create images, an MRI is not for patients with implanted hardware (e.g., pacemakers, etc.) or pregnant women.

27.24 Single Photon Emission Computed Tomography (SPECT)

Single photon emission computed tomography (SPECT) involves an intravenous injection of a radiopharmaceutical to enhance the image. It is done to detect cerebral blood flow, stroke, dementia, amnesia, neoplasm, head trauma, seizures, persistent vegetative state, brain death, and psychiatric disorders. This test is not for pregnant women.

Solved Problems

Nervous System

27.1 What is a concussion?

A concussion involves a blow to the head in which there is a bruising-type injury as the brain is thrust against the inside of skull. The point of injury where the brain makes impact against the skull is referred to as a coup injury.

27.2 What is amyotrophic lateral sclerosis (ALS)?

ALS is commonly called Lou Gehrig's disease and is a progressive, degenerative disorder that involves both the upper and lower motor neurons.

27.3 How does ALS affect the sensory function of the patient?

There is no change in mental status or sensory function with the disease. The disease does result in paralysis of the motor system, except the eyes.

27.4 What is Bell's palsy?

This is an acute idiopathic facial paralysis of the seventh cranial nerve that affects one side of the face.

27.5 What is a brain abscess?

A brain abscess is a collection of pus that creates a space-occupying area within the brain.

27.6 What is a cerebral aneurysm?

A cerebral aneurysm is a balloon-like outpouching caused by a congenital or developed weakness in a cerebral artery.

27.7 What might cause a cerebral aneurysm?

Trauma, infection, or vessel wall lesions caused by atherosclerosis can all lead to the development of an aneurysm. Increased pressure within the vessel lumen may cause the aneurysm to rupture, causing significant intracranial bleeding.

27.8 What is encephalitis?

Encephalitis is inflammation of the brain tissue, most often caused by a virus, although it can also be caused by bacteria, fungus, or protozoa.

27.9 What is viral encephalitis?

In the case of viral encephalitis, the patient typically will have had viral symptoms before the current illness. The virus enters the CNS via the bloodstream and begins to reproduce. Inflammation in the area follows, causing damage to the neurons.

27.10 What is Guillain-Barré syndrome?

This is an acute, progressive autoimmune condition that affects the peripheral nerves. Symptoms occur as the myelin surrounding the axon on the peripheral nerves is damaged from the autoimmune effect. The disease typically follows a viral infection, surgery, other acute illness or immunization by a couple of weeks.

27.11 What is ascending Guillain-Barré?

Ascending Guillain-Barré exhibits muscle weakness and/or paralysis that begins in the distal lower extremities and travels upward.

27.12 What is descending Guillain-Barré?

Descending Guillain-Barré begins with muscles in the face, jaw, or throat and travels downward.

27.13 What is Huntington's disease?

This is a degenerative disease that presents with a gradual onset of involuntary, jerking movements (chorea) and a progressive decline in mental ability, resulting in behavioral changes and dementia.

27.14 What is meningitis?

Meningitis is the inflammation of the meningeal coverings of the brain and spinal cord, most commonly caused by bacteria or virus, although it can also be caused by fungus, protozoa, or toxic exposure.

27.15 What is multiple sclerosis?

This is an autoimmune disease that results in demyelination of the white matter of the nervous system. Nerve impulses travel along the myelin coating on the outside of the nerve cells. With the disruption in the myelin on the outside of the nerve cells, the transmission of information from cell to cell within the nervous system is altered.

27.16 What is myasthenia gravis?

This is a disorder of the PNS involving antibodies that have been produced by the body; they bind to receptor sites that normally bind acetylcholine. This prevents the acetylcholine from binding to the receptor sites on the skeletal muscle, causing abnormal muscle contraction in the affected area.

27.17 What is Parkinson's disease?

There is a gradual degeneration of the midbrain area known as the substantia nigra. The neurons use the neurotransmitter dopamine to send their signals from cell to cell. The loss of neurons within the substantia nigra continues and results in diminished voluntary fine motor skills due to dopamine loss. There is also development of sympathetic noradrenergic lesions, causing norepinephrine loss within the sympathetic nervous system.

27.18 When is permanent injury assessed in a spinal cord injury?

Swelling caused by the initial trauma may make the injury seem more severe than it actually is. When the initial swelling resolves, the actual degree of permanent injury can be more accurately assessed.

27.19 What is a stroke?

A stroke is also known as a cerebrovascular accident (CVA) or brain attack. Blood supply is interrupted to part of the brain, causing brain cells to die. This results in the patient losing brain function in the affected area.

27.20 What is a seizure disorder?

This is a disorder that involves a sudden episode of abnormal, uncontrolled discharge of the electrical activity of the neurons within the brain. The patient may experience a variety of symptoms depending on the type of seizure and the cause.

27.21 What causes a seizure?

Seizures may be a symptom of another condition—such as a tumor or stroke that has increased the intracranial pressure, a metabolic disorder, withdrawal from alcohol or drugs—or may be caused by a chronic seizure disorder such as epilepsy.

27.22 What is the purpose of the SPECT?

SPECT involves an intravenous injection of a radiopharmaceutical to enhance the image. It is done to detect cerebral blood flow, stroke, dementia, amnesia, neoplasm, head trauma, seizures, persistent vegetative state, brain death, and psychiatric disorders

27.23 What is the purpose of an MRI with gadolinium?

This test is done to detect differences in tissue integrity, tumors, and disc disease.

27.24 Why is an electronystagmogram administered?

An electronystagmogram assesses the underlying cause of loss of balance and vertigo.

27.25 What is a lumbar puncture?

A spinal needle is inserted into the subarachnoid space at the levels of L3–L4 or L4–L5 with the patient lying on his or her side with knees drawn up to the chest. This test is performed under local anesthesia. It is done to obtain pressure readings, obtain cerebrospinal fluid for analysis, inject contrast material or air for diagnostic tests, inject medications, or reduce increased intracranial pressure.

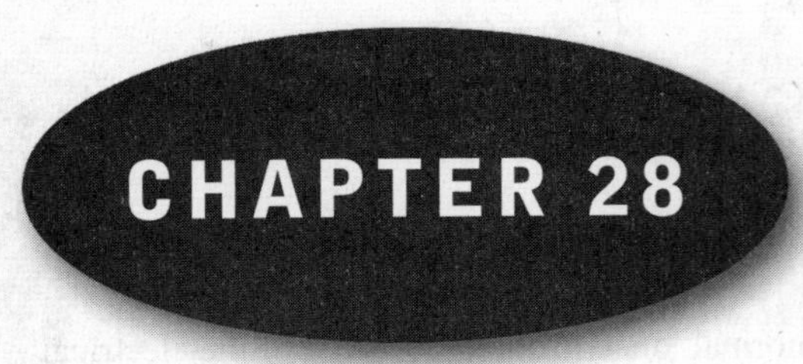

The Musculoskeletal System

28.1 Definition

The musculoskeletal system provides both structure and function for the body. The bones protect and support the vital organs. The skeleton is divided into the axial and appendicular areas. The axial skeleton protects the vital organs, surrounding the central nervous system (CNS) and thoracic cavity. The appendicular skeleton attaches to the axial skeleton and consists primarily of the limbs.

Bones are classified by both their shape and their composition. Short bones (like the phalanges) are found in the fingers and toes. Long bones (like the humerus or femur) are found in the limbs. Irregular bones are named for their shapes and are found in the joints of the ankle or wrist and in the middle ear.

Flat bones (ribs or scapula) protect inner organs. The outer layer of bone tissue is a dense compact bone tissue called the cortex.

Blood supply for the bone travels through small blood vessels within haversian canals located longitudinally within the cortical bone area. The inner layer is spongier, cancellous tissue that has spaces filled with marrow. Production of blood cells occurs within the red bone marrow. Yellow bone marrow is composed primarily of fat cells.

Osteoblasts (bone-building cells) and osteoclasts (bone-resorbing cells) are found in the outer layer of the bone. Joints are the areas in which two or more bones come together. Joints are described as being freely movable (synovial joints like the hip), partially movable (pelvic bones), or immovable (suture lines in the skull).

Synovial joints are lined with synovium. This membrane secretes synovial fluid to lubricate the joint and act as a shock absorber during motion or weight bearing. Synovial joints have a variety of range of motion, including flexion, extension, rotation, circumduction, supination, pronation, abduction, adduction, inversion, and eversion.

Partially movable joints have specific small amounts of motion that are typical of the joint space. Pelvic bones and individual joints between the vertebral bones are partially movable. Immovable joints are areas in which bones come together, but no movement is allowed. Muscles work in groups, with one set of muscles relaxing as another set contracts to create motion. A small amount of muscle contraction is typical to maintain muscle tone within the muscles.

Skeletal muscle is striated and voluntary. Connective tissues are the pieces that hold other parts together. Tendons attach muscles to bones; ligaments attach bones to bones. Cartilage provides a smooth surface within joints to ease movement and provide cushioning to weight-bearing joints. Bursa are small fluid-filled sacs, within joint areas or adjacent to bone, that provide cushioning at points of friction.

28.2 Carpal Tunnel Syndrome

The median nerve that passes through the carpal tunnel in the anterior wrist is compressed, resulting in pain and a numb sensation to the thumb, and index finger, middle finger, and lateral aspect of the fourth finger in the hand. This is often the result of repetitive hand motions and may be related to work or hobbies. Carpal tunnel syndrome tends to be more common in women.

28.3 Fractures

Excess stress or direct trauma is placed on a bone, causing a break. This results in damage to surrounding muscles and tissue, leading to hemorrhage, edema, and local tissue damage. Initially after the fracture, bleeding in the area leads to hematoma formation at the site. Inflammatory cells enter the area. Granulation tissue replaces the hematoma. Cellular changes continue and a nonbony union known as a callus develops. Osteoblasts continue to enter the area. Fibrous tissue in the fractured area changes to bone. The fracture site may be just a crack in the bone, without displacing any of the bone itself.

A fracture that does not go all the way through the bone is considered an incomplete fracture. The fracture may also go all the way through a bone, breaking it into two (or more) pieces, which is referred to as a complete fracture.

The surrounding muscle tissue that attaches above and below the fracture area in a limb will continue to create tension on their attachment points to the bone and pull the pieces further out of alignment. Some fractured bone pieces may penetrate through the skin; this is known as an open or compound fracture. Those that do not penetrate the skin are considered closed or simple fractures.

28.4 Gout

Gout is a metabolic disorder in which the body does not properly metabolize purine-based proteins. As a result, there is an increase in the amount of uric acid, which is the end product of purine metabolism.

As a result of hyperuricemia, uric acid crystals accumulate in joints, most commonly the big toe (podagra), causing pain when the joint moves. Uric acid is cleared from the body through the kidneys. These patients may also develop kidney stones as the uric acid crystallizes in the kidney.

A person may also develop secondary gout. This is caused by another disease process or use of medication, such as thiazide diuretics or some chemotherapeutic agents.

28.5 Osteoarthritis

Osteoarthritis is a degenerative joint disease caused by the wear and tear of the articular cartilage. As the protective joint cartilage is worn away, the underlying bone becomes exposed, causing the exposed bones to rub.

Degenerative changes within the bone tissue produce small areas of regrowth, causing jagged joint spaces and bone spurs. These rough areas project out into soft tissue or joint spaces, causing pain.

28.6 Osteomyelitis

Osteomyelitis is an infection of the bone. In an adult, it is most commonly caused by direct contamination of the site during trauma, such as an open fracture. Bacteria that cause infections elsewhere in the body may also enter the bloodstream and become deposited into the bone, starting a secondary infection site there.

This is more common in children and adolescents. Some of the patients have been treated with antibiotics previously for the initial infection. The causative organism is not always identified.

More than three-fourths of the identified organisms are *Staphylococcus aureus*. Acute infection is associated with inflammatory changes in the bone and may lead to necrosis. Some patients develop chronic osteomyelitis.

28.7 Osteoporosis

Osteoporosis is a decrease in bone density, making bones more brittle and increasing the risk of fracture. The body continuously replaces older bone with new bone through a balance between osteoblastic and osteoclastic activity.

When bone-building activity does not keep up with bone-resorption activity, the structural integrity of the bone is compromised. Increased age, lack of physical activity, poor nutrition, having a small frame, and being Caucasian, Asian, or female all increase the risk of osteoporosis.

Osteoporosis can also occur as a secondary disease, because of another condition. These causes include use of medications such as corticosteroids or some anticonvulsants, hormonal disorders (e.g., Cushing's or thyroid), and prolonged immobilization.

28.8 Arthrogram

An X-ray of a joint area is taken after the injection of a contrast material has been injected into the joint space to enhance its visibility. In a double-contrast study, a solution is injected, followed by air. This may be done to better assess the possibility of bone chips or torn ligaments within the joint space.

28.9 Arthroscopy

Arthroscopy is a fiberoptic scope used to visually examine the joint, performed under some type of anesthesia (local, epidural, conscious sedation, or general). This is done to perform surgery concurrently, diagnose injuries to joint spaces, and assess response to prior treatments.

28.10 Bone Scan

This is a peripheral intravenous injection of a bone-seeking radiopharmaceutical followed by a 2- to 3-hour delayed imaging. The patient must lie still for the duration of the scanning, about 30 to 60 minutes. It is done to diagnose osteomyelitis, bone tumors, metastatic disease, fractures, and unexplained skeletal pain.

The practitioner should encourage fluids after the injection to flush the radiopharmaceutical. The practitioner should also monitor for reaction to the radiopharmaceutical: rash, itching, hives. Computed tomography (CT) scan and computerized axial tomography (computer-manipulated pictures of radiologic images) should not be obstructed by overlying anatomy.

The patient must lie still during the exam for clear images. This is done to detect fractures and bone metastasis.

28.11 Electromyography (EMG)

Multiple small needle-type electrodes are inserted into muscle areas to test muscle potential. The patient may be asked to move the area to allow for measurement during minimal and maximal contraction of the muscle. The amount of muscle and nerve activity is recorded graphically.

There may be some discomfort during the testing. Certain medications may need to be stopped before testing: muscle relaxants, stimulants, caffeine. After the testing, the patient may complain of pain or anxiety. The test is done to detect neuromuscular, peripheral nerve disorders, or lower motor neuron disorders, and may be done in conjunction with nerve conduction studies.

Solved Problems

Musculoskeletal System

28.1 What is the function of the axial skeleton?

The axial skeleton protects the vital organs, surrounding the central nervous system and thoracic cavity.

28.2 What is the purpose of flat bones?

Flat bones (ribs or scapula) protect inner organs.

28.3 What are haversian canals?

Blood supply for the bone travels through small blood vessels within haversian canals located longitudinally within the cortical bone area.

28.4 Where are blood cells produced?

Production of blood cells occurs within the red bone marrow.

28.5 What are osteoblasts?

Osteoblasts are bone-building cells.

28.6 What are osteoclasts?

Osteoclasts are bone-resorbing cells.

28.7 What is synovium?

Synovial joints are lined with synovium. This membrane secretes synovial fluid to lubricate the joint and act as a shock absorber during motion or weight bearing.

28.8 Where is bone marrow located?

Within the cortical bone area, there is an inner layer of more spongy, cancellous tissue that has spaces filled with marrow.

28.9 How do muscles work with bone?

Muscles work in groups, with one set of muscles relaxing as another set contracts to create motion. A small amount of muscle contraction is typical to maintain muscle tone within the muscles.

28.10 What are tendons?

Tendons attach muscles to bones.

28.11 What are ligaments?

Ligaments attach bones to bones.

28.12 What is cartilage?

Cartilage provides a smooth surface within joints to ease movement and provide cushioning to weight-bearing joints.

28.13 What are bursa?

Bursa are small fluid-filled sacs, within joint areas or adjacent to bone that provide cushioning at points of friction.

28.14 What is carpal tunnel syndrome?

The median nerve that passes through the carpal tunnel in the anterior wrist is compressed, resulting in pain and a numb sensation to the thumb, and index finger, middle finger, and lateral aspect of the fourth finger in the hand.

28.15 What is a callus?

Initially after the fracture, bleeding in the area leads to hematoma formation at the site. Inflammatory cells enter the area. Granulation tissue replaces the hematoma. Cellular changes continue and a nonbony union known as a callus develops. Osteoblasts continue to enter the area. Fibrous tissue in the fractured area changes to bone.

28.16 What is an incomplete fracture?

A fracture that does not go all the way through the bone is considered an incomplete fracture.

28.17 What is a compound fracture?

Some fractured bone pieces may penetrate through the skin; this is known as an open or compound fracture.

28.18 What is a simple fracture?

Those that do not penetrate the skin are considered closed or simple fractures.

28.19 What is gout?

Gout is a metabolic disorder in which the body does not properly metabolize purine-based proteins. As a result, there is an increase in the amount of uric acid, which is the end product of purine metabolism.

28.20 What is osteoarthritis?

This is a degenerative joint disease caused by the wear and tear of the articular cartilage. As the protective joint cartilage is worn away, the underlying bone becomes exposed, causing the exposed bones to rub.

28.21 What is osteomyelitis?

Osteomyelitis is an infection of the bone.

28.22 What is a common cause of osteomyelitis in adults?

In an adult, it is most commonly caused by direct contamination of the site during trauma such as an open fracture. Bacteria that cause infections elsewhere in the body may also enter the bloodstream and become deposited in the bone, starting a secondary infection site there.

28.23 What is osteoporosis?

Osteoporosis is a decrease in bone density, making bones more brittle and increasing the risk of fracture. The body continuously replaces older bone with new bone through a balance between the osteoblastic and osteoclastic activity.

28.24 What is an arthrogram?

An X-ray of a joint area is taken after the injection of a contrast material has been injected into the joint space to enhance its visibility. In a double-contrast study, a solution is injected, followed by air. This may be done to better assess the possibility of bone chips or torn ligaments within the joint space.

28.25 What is a confrontation test?

This test assesses the patient's peripheral vision by gazing at the health care provider's nose.

The Gastrointestinal System

29.1 Definition

The gastrointestinal system includes the alimentary canal (mouth, esophagus, stomach, small intestine, large intestine, and rectum), accessory organs (salivary glands, liver, pancreas, and gallbladder), and ducts.

The alimentary canal is a hollow tube lined with mucous membrane. The gastrointestinal tract functions to digest food, absorb nutrients, propel the contents through the lumen, and eliminate the waste products. Digestion of food has both mechanical and chemical components. Both processes begin in the mouth. Chewing, movement through the gastrointestinal (GI) tract, and churning within the stomach are parts of the mechanical process. Saliva, hydrochloric acid, bile, and other digestive enzymes all contribute to the chemical process of digestion.

The esophagus extends from the oropharynx to the stomach. At the top of the esophagus is the upper esophageal sphincter (UES) to prevent the influx of air into the esophagus during respiration. At the bottom of the esophagus is the lower esophageal sphincter (LES) to prevent the reflux of acid from the stomach into the esophagus. The contents of the esophagus empty into the stomach through the cardiac sphincter. The stomach secretes gastrin, which promotes secretion of pepsinogen and hydrochloric acid, pepsin, and lipase, all of which aid digestion, and mucus formation, which helps protect the stomach lining.

The liver is a very vascular organ located in the right upper quadrant of the abdomen under the diaphragm. It has two main lobes that are comprised of smaller lobules. The liver stores a variety of vitamins and minerals. It metabolizes proteins; synthesizes plasma proteins, fatty acids, and triglycerides; and stores and releases glycogen.

The liver detoxifies foreign substances such as alcohol, drugs, or chemicals. The liver forms and secretes bile to aid in digestion of fat. Bile releases into the gallbladder for storage or into the duodenum if needed for digestion if the sphincter of Oddi is open because of secretion of the digestive enzymes secretin, cholecystokinin, and gastrin.

The gallbladder is a small receptacle that holds bile until it is needed. It is located on the inferior aspect of the liver. The pancreas is located retroperitoneally in the upper abdomen near the stomach and extends from just right of midline to the left toward the spleen.

The pancreas has both endocrine and exocrine functions. The endocrine functions include secretion of insulin in response to elevations in blood glucose from the beta cells of the islets of Langerhans and glucagon in response to decrease in blood glucose from the alpha cells. The exocrine function includes secretion of trypsin, lipase, amylase, and chymotrypsin to aid in digestion.

The small intestine is composed of the duodenum, jejunum, and ileum. The duodenum attaches to the stomach, is about 1 foot long and C-shaped, and curves to the left around the pancreas. The common bile duct and pancreatic duct enter here. The jejunum is between the duodenum and ileum and is about 8 feet long.

The last portion of the small intestine is the ileum, which is up to 12 feet long, depending on the size of the patient. The ileocecal valve separates the ileum from the large intestine. The appendix is found at this juncture.

The large intestine can be broken down into the ascending colon, transverse colon, descending colon, and sigmoid colon. The sigmoid colon joins the rectum and ultimately the anal canal.

29.2 Appendicitis

Inflammation of the vermiform appendix (a blind pouch located near the ileocecal valve in the right lower quadrant of the abdomen) is known as appendicitis. It may be caused by obstruction from stool.

The mucosal lining of the appendix continues to secrete fluid, which increases the pressure within the lumen of the appendix, causing a restriction of the blood supply to the appendix. This decrease in blood supply may result in gangrene or perforation as the pressure continues to build. Pain localizes at McBurney's point, located midway between the umbilicus and right anterior iliac crest. Appendicitis may occur at any age, but the peak occurrence is from the teenage years to age 30.

29.3 Cholecystitis

An inflammation of the gallbladder, often accompanied by the formation of gallstones (cholelithiasis), is cholecystitis. The inflammation may be either acute or chronic in nature. In an acute cholecystitis, the blood flow to the gallbladder may become compromised, which in turn causes problems with the normal filling and emptying of the gallbladder. A stone may block the cystic duct, which results in bile becoming trapped within the gallbladder because of inflammation around the stone within the duct.

Blood flow to the inflamed area is minimized, localized edema develops, the gallbladder distends because of retained bile, and ischemic changes occur within the wall of the gallbladder. Chronic cholecystitis occurs when there have been recurrent episodes of blockage of the cystic duct, usually because of stones. There is chronic inflammation.

The gallbladder is often contracted, which leads to problems with storing and moving the bile. Patients may develop jaundice because of a backup of bile or obstructive jaundice. They exhibit a yellowish tone to skin and mucous membranes. If patients have a naturally dark pigmentation to their skin, the practitioner should check palms and soles.

Icterus is the yellow color change seen in the sclera (white) of the eye. There is increased risk for gallbladder inflammation and development of gallstones with increasing age, being female or overweight, having a family history, people on rapid weight loss diets, and during pregnancy.

29.4 Cirrhosis

Injury to the cellular structure of the liver causes fibrosis because of chronic inflammation and necrotic changes, resulting in cirrhosis. There are nodular changes to the liver. The bile ducts and blood vessels through the liver may become blocked because of both the nodular changes and fibrosis.

These changes to the liver cause enlargement of the organ and change in texture. There is increased pressure within the portal vein. This causes resistance to blood flow throughout the venous system in the liver and also backs up venous blood to the spleen, causing enlargement of this organ also.

Damage to the liver may be reversible if the cause is identified early and removed. The most common causes of cirrhosis include chronic alcohol use, liver damage secondary to exposure to drugs or toxins, viral hepatitis (especially hepatitis B, hepatitis C, and hepatitis D in those already infected with hepatitis B), fatty liver (steatohepatitis), autoimmune hepatitis, cystic fibrosis, metabolic disorders (excess iron storage—hemochromatosis), or genetic causes.

29.5 Crohn's Disease

Crohn's disease is a noncontinuous inflammatory disease that can affect any point from the mouth to the anus. The majority of cases involve the small and large intestine, often in the right lower quadrant at the point where the terminal ileum and the ascending colon meet.

Patients typically have an insidious onset of intermittent symptoms. The disease causes transmural inflammation, going deeper than the superficial mucosal layer of the tissue to affect all layers. Over time the inflammatory changes within the GI tract can lead to strictures or the formation of fistulas. The affected tissue develops granulomas and takes on a mottled appearance interspersed with normal tissue. There is a genetic predisposition.

29.6 Diverticulitis

Small outpouchings called diverticula develop along the intestinal tract. Diverticulosis is the condition of having these diverticula. Any part of the large or small intestine may be involved. The area of the intestinal tract that most commonly develops diverticula is the lower portion of the large intestine. Certain types of undigested foods can become trapped in the pouches of the intestine.

Bacteria multiply in the area, causing further inflammation. Diverticulitis is an inflammation of at least one of the diverticula. Diets that have a low fiber content, seeds, or nuts have been implicated in the development of diverticulitis. Perforation of the diverticula is possible when they are inflamed.

29.7 Gastroenteritis

This is an acute inflammation of the gastric and intestinal mucosa that is most commonly caused by bacterial, viral, protozoal, or parasitic infection. It may also be caused by irritation due to chemical or toxin exposure or allergic response. Viral exposure is more likely in winter; bacterial exposure is more common in winter when foodborne illness exposure is likely.

29.8 Gastroesophageal Reflux Disease (GERD)

Gastroesophageal reflux disease (GERD) is the reflux of stomach acid and contents into the esophagus. This typically causes symptoms because the lining of the esophagus is not protected against the acid that is normally found only in the stomach. The pain that is produced is often referred to as heartburn, or may be mistaken for cardiac pain. The pain may also extend to the back.

The pain occurs more frequently in men, people who are obese, smokers, and those who use alcohol or medications that lower the muscle tone of the lower esophageal sphincter. The pain caused by acid refluxing into the esophagus is worse after eating or when lying down. Patients with a hiatal hernia may also experience reflux because of the increased pressure that exists from a portion of the stomach protruding upward through the diaphragm.

29.9 Gastrointestinal Bleeds

Bleeding from the GI tract may cause significant blood loss. The bleeding may be from either the upper or lower GI tract. Upper gastrointestinal bleeds are commonly from ulcers, esophageal varices, neoplasms, arteriovenous malformations, Mallory-Weiss tears secondary to vomiting, or anticoagulant use.

Lower gastrointestinal bleeds are commonly caused by fissure formation, rectal trauma, colitis, polyps, colon cancer, diverticulitis, vasculitis, or ulcerations.

29.10 Gastritis

Gastritis is an inflammation of the stomach lining resulting from either erosive or atrophic causes. Erosive causes include stresses such as physical illness or medications such as nonsteroidal anti-inflammatory drugs (NSAIDs). Atrophic causes include a history of prior surgery (such as gastrectomy), pernicious anemia, alcohol use, or *Helicobacter pylori* infection.

29.11 Hepatitis

Hepatitis is an inflammation of the liver cells. This most commonly results from a viral cause, which may be either an acute illness or become chronic. The disease may also be caused by exposure to drugs or toxins.

- **Hepatitis A:** Hepatitis A is transmitted via an oral route, often by contaminated water or poor sanitation when traveling; it is also transmitted in daycare settings and residential institutions. It can be prevented by vaccine.
- **Hepatitis B:** Hepatitis B is transmitted via a percutaneous route, often by sexual contact, IV drug use, mother-to-neonate transmission, or possibly blood transfusion. It can be prevented by vaccine.
- **Hepatitis C:** Hepatitis C is transmitted via a percutaneous route, often by IV drug use or, less commonly, sexual contact. There is currently no vaccine available.
- **Hepatitis D:** Hepatitis D is transmitted via a percutaneous route and needs hepatitis B to spread cell to cell. There is no vaccine available for hepatitis D.
- **Hepatitis E:** Hepatitis E is transmitted via an oral route and is associated with water contamination. There is no known chronic state of hepatitis E and no current vaccine available.
- **Hepatitis G:** Hepatitis G is transmitted via a percutaneous route and is associated with chronic infection but not significant liver disease.

Exposure to medications (even at therapeutic doses), drugs, or chemicals can also cause hepatitis. Onset is usually within the first couple of days of use, and may be within the first couple of doses. Hepatotoxic substances include acetaminophen, carbon tetrachloride, benzenes, and valproic acid.

29.12 Hiatal Hernia

This is also known as a diaphragmatic hernia. A part of the stomach protrudes up through the diaphragm near the esophagus into the chest. Patients may be asymptomatic or have daily symptoms of gastroesophageal reflux disease (GERD).

The hernia may be a sliding hiatal hernia, which allows movement of the upper portion of the stomach including the lower esophageal sphincter up and down through the diaphragm. These patients typically have symptoms of GERD.

Another type of hiatal hernia is a rolling hernia, in which a portion of the stomach protrudes up through the diaphragm, but the lower esophageal sphincter area remains below the level of the diaphragm. These patients do not generally suffer from reflux.

29.13 Intestinal Obstruction and Paralytic Ileus

An intestinal obstruction occurs when motility through the intestine is blocked. This may be caused by a mechanical obstruction due to the presence of a tumor, adhesions from prior surgery, or infection or fecal impaction.

A paralytic ileus results when motility through the intestine is blocked without any obstructing mass. This may occur during the postoperative period following intraabdominal surgery, during a severe systemic illness (sepsis), electrolyte imbalance, or because of a metabolic disorder (diabetic ketoacidosis).

29.14 Pancreatitis

Pancreatitis is an inflammation of the pancreas that causes destructive cellular changes. It may be an acute or a chronic process. Acute pancreatitis involves autodigestion of the pancreas by pancreatic enzymes and development of fibrosis. Blood glucose control may be affected by the changes to the pancreas.

Chronic pancreatitis results from recurrent episodes of exacerbation, leading to fibrosis and a decrease in pancreatic function. Presence of gallstones blocking a pancreatic duct, chronic use of alcohol, postabdominal trauma or surgery, or elevated cholesterol are associated with an increased risk of pancreatitis.

29.15 Peritonitis

Peritonitis is an acute inflammation of the peritoneum, which is the lining of the abdominal cavity. Peritonitis may be primary or secondary to another disease process. It typically occurs because of bacterial presence within the peritoneal space.

The bacteria may have passed from the GI tract or the rupture of an organ within the abdomen or pelvis. After the introduction of the bacteria into the abdominal area, an inflammatory reaction occurs.

29.16 Peptic Ulcer Disease (PUD)

An ulcer develops when there is erosion of a portion of the mucosal layer of either the stomach or duodenum. The ulcer may occur within the stomach (gastric ulcer) or the duodenum (duodenal ulcer). A break in the protective mucosal lining allows the acid within the stomach to make contact with the epithelial tissues. Gastric ulcers favor the lesser curvature of the stomach.

Duodenal ulcers tend to be deeper, penetrating through the mucosa to the muscular layer. *H. pylori* infection has been associated with duodenal ulcers. Stress ulcers are associated with another acute medical condition or traumatic injury.

As the body attempts to heal from the other physical condition (e.g., major surgery), small areas of ischemia develop within the stomach or duodenum. The ischemic areas then ulcerate.

29.17 Ulcerative Colitis

Ulcerative colitis is an inflammatory disease of the large intestine that affects the mucosal layer beginning in the rectum and colon and spreading into the adjacent tissue. There are ulcerations in the mucosal layer of the intestinal wall, and inflammation and abscess formation occur. Bloody diarrhea with mucus is the primary symptom.

There are periods of exacerbations and remissions. Symptom severity may vary from mild to severe. The exact cause is unknown, but there is increased incidence in people with northern European, North American, or

Ashkenazi Jewish origins. The peak incidences are from mid-teens to mid-20s and again from mid-50s to mid-60s.

29.18 Gastroscopy

This test is used to diagnose peptic, gastric, or duodenal ulcers and obtain biopsies and specimens for *H. pylori* bacteria. An informed consent is obtained before any anesthesia. An endoscope is passed through the mouth to allow visualization of the pharynx, esophagus, lower esophageal sphincter, stomach, pyloric sphincter, and duodenum.

Biopsies can be obtained at this time. Bleeding, ulcers, lesions, and polyps can be visually assessed. The back of the throat will be anesthetized to allow passage of the endoscope.

Before the Test: The patient is NPO (nothing by mouth).

After the Test: The practitioner should monitor vital signs and assess for return of gag reflex. The patient remains NPO until the gag reflex returns.

29.19 Colonoscopy

This test is used to diagnose obstruction, bleeding, change in bowel habits, and colon cancer, among other conditions. An informed consent is obtained before the patient is given any type of anesthesia.

A colonoscope is passed through the rectum to visualize the anus, sigmoid, descending colon, splenic flexure, transverse colon, hepatic flexure, ascending colon, and the ileocecal valve. The colon may be insufflated to aid in visualization of the structures.

Biopsies are obtained as indicated. The scope is withdrawn and anesthesia is reversed. The patient may experience abdominal distention. Risks include perforation of the large intestine. The test is commonly performed as an outpatient procedure.

Before the Test: A thorough colon prep is necessary to ensure complete emptying of the bowel before the procedure. The patient is NPO for several hours before the test because of the use of an anesthetic agent.

After the Test: The practitioner should assess the abdomen for bowel sounds and tenderness. Monitor vital signs. Assess the patient for side effects of anesthesia.

29.20 Abdominal Ultrasound

This is a noninvasive test and is usually painless. A transducer is guided over the abdomen, which produces sound waves that bounce off internal structures and produce a picture of internal organs and structures.

Before the Test: The patient needs to be NPO.

After the Test: No special care is needed.

29.21 Liver Biopsy

Here, a small sample of tissue is removed from the liver and examined under a microscope, allowing for a definite diagnosis. A thin, cutting needle, through the skin of the abdomen, is used to obtain the sample.

Needle biopsies are relatively simple procedures requiring only local anesthesia. Risks include bruising, bleeding, and infection.

Before the Test: Informed consent is needed.

After the Test: The practitioner should monitor vital signs for drop in blood pressure as well as an increase in pulse or respiration. The practitioner should check the site for bruising or bleeding, and check the skin for pallor or sweating.

29.22 Endoscopic Retrograde Cholangiopancreatography (ERCP)

Here, a thin, flexible tube (endoscope) is passed through the pharynx, the stomach, and into the upper part of the small intestine. Air is used to inflate the intestinal tract to enable the openings of the pancreatic and bile ducts to be seen. A dye is injected into the ducts through a catheter via the endoscope. X-rays are taken of the ducts. The patient may report abdominal distention from the insufflation and a sore throat.

Before the Test: The patient is NPO.

After the Test: The practitioner should monitor vital signs and assess for return of gag reflex. The patient remains NPO until gag reflex returns.

29.23 Liver Function Tests

These comprise several tests, obtained through a venipuncture, that show hepatic function. They generally include:

- **Alanine Transaminase (ALT):** An enzyme found mainly in liver cells, ALT helps the body metabolize protein. When the liver is damaged, ALT is released in the bloodstream.
- **Aspartate Transaminase (AST):** The enzyme AST plays a role in the metabolism of alanine, an amino acid. An increase in AST levels may indicate liver damage or disease.
- **Alkaline Phosphatase (ALP):** ALP is an enzyme found in high concentrations in the liver and bile ducts, as well as some other tissues. Higher-than-normal levels of ALP may indicate liver damage or disease.
- **Albumin and Total Protein:** Levels of albumin—a protein made by the liver—and total protein show how well the liver is making proteins that the body needs to fight infections and perform other functions. Lower-than-normal levels may indicate liver damage or disease.
- **Bilirubin:** Bilirubin is a red-yellow pigment that results from the breakdown of red blood cells. Normally, bilirubin passes through the liver and is excreted in stool. Elevated levels of bilirubin (jaundice) may indicate liver damage or disease.
- **Gamma-Glutamyl Transferase (GGT):** This test measures the amount of the enzyme GGT in the blood. Higher-than-normal levels may indicate liver or bile duct injury.
- **Lactate Dehydrogenase (LDH):** LDH is an enzyme found in many body tissues, including the liver. Elevated levels of LDH may indicate liver damage.
- **Prothrombin Time (PT):** This test measures the clotting time of plasma. Increased PT may indicate liver damage.
- **Hepatitis Panel:** Tests for acute viral hepatitis include HBsAg, anti-HAV, IgM anti-HBc, and anti-HCV. Tests for chronic hepatitis include HBsAg and anti-HCV. HAV is confirmed by detecting an IgM antibody to HAV (IgM anti-HAV); HBV by HBsAg and IgM anti-HBC (when HBeAg is detected, the patient is highly infectious); HCV by ELISA–2 and RIBA–2;

HDV by anti-HDV and serologic markers for HBV. For HEV, only research-based tests are available at this time.

Solved Problems

Gastrointestinal System

29.1 What is appendicitis?

Inflammation of the vermiform appendix (a blind pouch located near the ileocecal valve in the right lower quadrant of the abdomen) is known as appendicitis.

29.2 What is McBurney's point?

Pain from appendicitis localizes at McBurney's point, located midway between the umbilicus and right anterior iliac crest.

29.3 What is cholecystitis?

Cholecystitis is inflammation of the gallbladder.

29.4 What is acute cholecystitis?

In an acute cholecystitis, the blood flow to the gallbladder may become compromised, which in turn causes problems with the normal filling and emptying of the gallbladder. A stone may block the cystic duct, which results in bile becoming trapped within the gallbladder because of inflammation around the stone within the duct.

29.5 What is icterus?

Icterus is the yellow color change seen in the sclera (white) of the eye.

29.6 What is cirrhosis?

Injury to the cellular structure of the liver causes fibrosis because of chronic inflammation and necrotic changes, resulting in cirrhosis.

29.7 What are the common causes of cirrhosis?

The most common causes of cirrhosis include chronic alcohol use, liver damage secondary to exposure to drugs or toxins, viral hepatitis (especially hepatitis B, hepatitis C, and hepatitis D in those already infected with hepatitis B), fatty liver (steatohepatitis), autoimmune hepatitis, cystic fibrosis, metabolic disorders (excess iron storage—hemochromatosis), or genetic causes.

29.8 What is Crohn's disease?

Crohn's disease is a noncontinuous inflammatory disease that can affect any point from the mouth to the anus. The majority of cases involve the small and large intestines, often in the right lower quadrant at the point where the terminal ileum and the ascending colon meet.

29.9 What is diverticulitis disease?

Small outpouchings called diverticula develop along the intestinal tract. Diverticulosis is the condition of having these diverticula. Any part of the large or small intestine may be involved.

29.10 What is gastroenteritis?

Gastroenteritis is an acute inflammation of the gastric and intestinal mucosa and is most commonly caused by bacterial, viral, protozoal, or parasitic infection.

29.11 What is gastroesophageal reflux disease (GERD)?

GERD is the reflux of stomach acid and contents into the esophagus. This typically causes symptoms, because the lining of the esophagus is not protected against the acid that is normally found only in the stomach. The pain that is produced is often referred to as heartburn, or may be mistaken for cardiac pain.

29.12 What is gastritis?

Gastritis is an inflammation of the stomach lining resulting from either erosive or atrophic causes.

29.13 What is hepatitis?

Hepatitis is an inflammation of the liver cells.

29.14 What is a hiatal hernia?

This is also known as a diaphragmatic hernia. A part of the stomach protrudes up through the diaphragm near the esophagus into the chest.

29.15 What is a paralytic ileus?

A paralytic ileus results when motility through the intestine is blocked without any obstructing mass.

29.16 What might cause a paralytic ileus?

This may occur during the postoperative period following intraabdominal surgery, during a severe systemic illness (sepsis), electrolyte imbalance, or because of a metabolic disorder (diabetic ketoacidosis).

29.17 What is pancreatitis?

Pancreatitis is an inflammation of the pancreas that causes destructive cellular changes.

29.18 What is acute pancreatitis?

Acute pancreatitis involves autodigestion of the pancreas by pancreatic enzymes and development of fibrosis.

29.19 What is chronic pancreatitis?

Chronic pancreatitis results from recurrent episodes of exacerbation, leading to fibrosis and a decrease in pancreatic function.

29.20 What is peritonitis?

Peritonitis is an acute inflammation of the peritoneum, which is the lining of the abdominal cavity.

29.21 What is peptic ulcer disease (PUD)?

An ulcer develops when there is erosion of a portion of the mucosal layer of either the stomach or duodenum.

29.22 What is ulcerative colitis?

Ulcerative colitis is an inflammatory disease of the large intestine that affects the mucosal layer beginning in the rectum and colon and spreading into the adjacent tissue. There are ulcerations in the mucosal layer of the intestinal wall, and inflammation and abscess formation occur.

29.23 What is a sliding hiatal hernia?

A sliding hiatal hernia allows movement of the upper portion of the stomach including the lower esophageal sphincter up and down through the diaphragm. These patients typically have symptoms of GERD.

29.24 What is a rolling hernia?

A rolling hernia is a type of hiatal hernia in which a portion of the stomach protrudes up through the diaphragm, but the lower esophageal sphincter area remains below the level of the diaphragm. These patients do not generally suffer from reflux.

29.25 What are duodenal ulcers?

Duodenal ulcers are peptic ulcers that tend to be deeper, penetrating through the mucosa to the muscular layer. *H. pylori* infection has been associated with duodenal ulcers.

CHAPTER 30

The Endocrine System

30.1 Definition

The endocrine system is comprised of several glands, scattered throughout the body. The glands release hormones that are chemical messengers, substances that control and regulate the activity of target cells and organs.

Together, these hormones influence growth, development, and digestion, and regulate metabolism and reproduction. The glands generally release the hormones into the blood because of a stimulus, another hormone, or a threshold. The signal to turn off the hormone production is regulated by a process called direct feedback. Direct feedback is necessary to maintain homeostasis. The body receives feedback about changes in hormone levels and impacts organs or body systems to adjust the hormone production to tell the body to return to homeostasis. When the concentration of the substance reaches a threshold, the gland and its production are turned off. The glands, the hormones they produce, and the effects are discussed below.

The thyroid gland is located in the anterior neck, overlying the trachea. It makes three hormones: thyroxine (T4), triiodothyronine (T3), and calcitonin, which affects the blood calcium and phosphate release from the bones. Thyroid hormones affect metabolism, muscles, the heart, and many other body organs and systems. They help regulate carbohydrate metabolism, lipids, proteins, and growth and development.

Anterior pituitary glands are controlled by hormones from the hypothyroid and direct feedback.

The adrenal glands are bilateral glands that cap each kidney. They are located in the retroperitoneum. The glands are composed of two parts: the cortex and the adrenal medulla. The cortex secretes (1) aldosterone, which is responsible for renal reabsorption of sodium and excretion of potassium; (2) cortisol, which maintains glucose control, increases hepatic gluconeogenesis (the making of glucose), and manages the body's stress response; and (3) androgens, which are sex hormones. The adrenal medulla produces, stores, and secretes epinephrine and norepinephrine, which are called catecholamines. When they are released, heart and respiratory rates increase, blood pressure rises, airways dilate, and an increase in the metabolic rate is seen.

The parathyroid glands are composed of usually four, but sometimes six or more small glands that are found on the posterior side of the thyroid gland. Their function is to produce parathyroid hormone (PTH). Parathyroid hormone maintains the calcium level in the blood. It also regulates the phosphorus level in the body. If the serum calcium level falls, PTH is released, which causes bones to break down, releasing calcium into the blood. It also causes the kidneys to decrease the calcium released in the urine, and increases phosphate excretion.

30.2 Hypothyroidism (Myxedema)

Hypothyroidism is a lack of, or too little, thyroid hormone commonly caused by Hashimoto's thyroiditis. Hashimoto's thyroiditis is a chronic disorder caused by abnormal antibodies that attack the thyroid gland. Hypothyroidism can also be caused by decreased production of the thyroid-stimlating hormone (TSH) from the pituitary gland, a side effect of surgery, inflammation of the thyroid gland, and treatment for hyperthyroidism.

30.3 Hyperthyroidism (Graves' Disease)

This is an overproduction of T3 and T4 by the thyroid gland that can be caused by an autoimmune disease in which the body's immune system attacks the thyroid gland. Other causes can be a benign tumor (adenoma), resulting in an enlarged thyroid gland (goiter), or an overproduction of thyroid-stimulating hormone (TSH) by the pituitary gland, caused by a pituitary tumor.

30.4 Simple Goiter

A lack of iodine in the patient's diet (endemic, simple goiter) causes the thyroid gland to become enlarged. This is seen less today because iodine is added to table salt. The thyroid gland can also become enlarged by ingesting large amounts of goitrogenic drugs or goitrogenic foods that decrease production of thyroxine (goitrogenic), such as strawberries, cabbage, peanuts, peas, peaches, and spinach. This results in sporadic simple goiter. A simple goiter is not caused by inflammation or neoplasm.

30.5 Hypopituitarism

Hypopituitarism results when the pituitary gland is unable to secrete a normal amount of pituitary hormones. Primary causes are pituitary tumors, inadequate blood supply to the pituitary gland, infection, radiation therapy, or surgical removal of a portion of the pituitary gland. Secondary causes affect the hypothalamus, which regulates the pituitary gland.

30.6 Hyperpituitarism (Acromegaly and Gigantism)

The pituitary gland produces an excessive amount of growth hormone. If hyperpituitarism occurs before epiphyseal closure, the patient (infants and children) has gigantism, resulting in an overgrowth of all body tissues. If hyperpituitarism occurs after epiphyseal closure, which is rare, the patient has acromegaly, resulting in bone thickening, growth in width (transverse growth), and enlarged organs (visceromegaly).

30.7 Hyperprolactinemia

This is an overproduction of the prolactin hormone that promotes lactation. Excessive secretion is usually caused by a pituitary tumor (prolactinoma) and may also be caused by hypothyroidism, chronic kidney disease, and medications that affect the pituitary gland.

30.8 Diabetes Insipidus

Either a decrease in antidiuretic hormone (ADH) production by the hypothalamus or the increased ADH by the pituitary gland causes a decreased ability of the kidneys to concentrate urine. This results in the excretion of large amounts of diluted urine. The patient then drinks large amounts of fluid to replace the increased urine output.

30.9 Syndrome of Inappropriate Secretion of Antidiuretic Hormone (SIADH)

The syndrome of inappropriate secretion of antidiuretic hormone (SIADH) is caused by too much ADH being secreted by the posterior pituitary gland. Antidiuretic hormone (ADH) is responsible for controlling the amount of water reabsorbed by the kidney; it prevents the loss of too much fluid. When too much water is detected, ADH production or secretion is halted. SIADH may be caused by damage to the hypothalamus or pituitary, inflammation of the brain, some medications such as selective serotonin reuptake inhibitors (SSRIs), carbamazepine, cyclophosphamides, and chlorpropamide. Certain cancers, especially lung, may produce ADH.

30.10 Addison's Disease

Addison's disease is inadequate secretion of corticosteroids from the adrenal cortex, resulting from damage to the adrenal cortex. Autoimmune destruction of the adrenal gland and tuberculosis are two common causes of Addison's disease. A patient can experience Addisonian crisis when infection, surgery, or other stressful events result in a decrease in the production of cortisol and aldosterone. Addisonian crisis is a medical emergency.

30.11 Cushing's Syndrome

The adrenal cortex secretes an excess of glucocorticoids or the pituitary gland an excess of adrenocorticotropic hormone (ACTH) as a result of a pituitary tumor, adrenal tumor, or from ongoing glucocorticoid therapy.

30.12 Primary Aldosteronism (Conn's Syndrome)

The adrenal cortex is secreting an excessive amount of aldosterone caused by an adrenal tumor, a malfunctioning adrenal cortex, or sources outside the adrenal gland producing aldosterone. Some medications such as calcium channel blockers can lower aldosterone levels, which can confuse the diagnosis.

30.13 Pheochromocytoma

A tumor on the adrenal medulla secretes excessive amounts of epinephrine and norepinephrine.

30.14 Hypoparathyroidism

Hypoparathyroidism is diminished functioning of the parathyroid glands leading to low levels of parathyroid hormone (PTH), which causes hypocalcemia. The primary cause of hypoparathyroidism is destruction of the glands by an autoimmune cause. Parathyroidectomy is no longer a major cause, since surgery now removes only the gland that is malfunctioning. Occasionally the gland(s) may be accidentally removed during thyroidectomy.

30.15 Hyperparathyroidism

Overactivity of the parathyroid glands caused by a tumor produces too much PTH, resulting in hypercalcemia and hypophosphatemia. Excess calcium is reabsorbed by the kidneys and may result in kidney stones; however, malfunction in the feedback mechanism prevents detection of excessive calcium levels in the blood, thereby failing to adjust the secretion of PTH. Parathyroid tumors are usually benign.

30.16 Diabetes Mellitus

Our body converts certain foods into glucose, which is the body's primary energy supply. Insulin from the beta cells of the pancreas is necessary to transport glucose into cells where it is used for cell metabolism. Diabetes mellitus occurs when beta cells either are unable to produce insulin (type I diabetes mellitus) or produce an insufficient amount of insulin (type II diabetes mellitus).

As a result, glucose does not enter cells but remains in the blood. Increased glucose levels in the blood signal to the patient to increase intake of fluid in an effort to flush glucose out of the body in urine. Patients then experience increased thirst and urination.

Cells become starved for energy because of the lack of glucose and signal to the patient to eat, causing the patient to experience an increase in hunger. There are three types of diabetes mellitus: (1) type I, known as insulin-dependent (IDDM), where beta cells are destroyed by an autoimmune process; (2) type II, known as non-insulin-dependent (NIDDM), where beta cells produce insufficient insulin; and (3) gestational diabetes mellitus, which occurs during pregnancy.

30.17 Metabolic Syndrome (Syndrome X/Dysmetabolic Syndrome)

These patients have a collection of symptoms that include high blood glucose, obesity, high blood pressure, and high triglycerides based on family history. Beta cells in the pancreas are unable to produce sufficient insulin; therefore, the liver produces a higher level of glucose. The patient is also insulin resistant. This syndrome leads to cardiovascular disease.

Solved Problems

Endocrine System

30.1 What are hormones?

Hormones are chemical messengers that control and regulate the activity of target cells and organs.

30.2 What is direct feedback?

Direct feedback is necessary to maintain homeostasis. The body receives feedback about changes in hormone levels and impacts organs or body systems to adjust the hormone production to tell the body to return to homeostasis.

30.3 What is calcitonin?

Calcitonin is a hormone released by the thyroid gland that affects the blood calcium and phosphate release from the bones.

30.4 What controls the anterior pituitary glands?

Anterior pituitary glands are controlled by hormones from the hypothyroid and direct feedback.

30.5 What is aldosterone?

Aldosterone is a hormone produced by the adrenal glands that is responsible for renal reabsorption of sodium and excretion of potassium.

30.6 What is cortisol?

Cortisol is a hormone produced by the adrenal glands that maintains glucose control, increases hepatic gluconeogenesis (the making of glucose), and manages the body's stress response.

30.7 What are catecholamines?

Catecholamines are a hormone produced by the adrenal glands that cause the heart and respiratory rates to increase, blood pressure to rise, airways to dilate, and the metabolic rate to increase.

30.8 What is the function of the parathyroid hormone?

The parathyroid hormone (PTH) maintains the calcium level in the blood. It also regulates the phosphorus level in the body.

30.9 What is myxedema?

Myxedema (hypothyroidism) is a lack of, or too little, thyroid hormone.

30.10 What is Hashimoto's thyroiditis?

Hashimoto's thyroiditis is a chronic disorder caused by abnormal antibodies that attack the thyroid gland. Hypothyroidism can also be caused by decreased production of TSH from the pituitary gland, a side effect of surgery, inflammation of the thyroid gland, and treatment for hyperthyroidism.

30.11 What is Graves' disease?

Graves' disease (hyperthyroidism) is an overproduction of T3 and T4 by the thyroid gland that can be caused by an autoimmune disease in which the body's immune system attacks the thyroid gland. Other causes can be a benign tumor (adenoma) resulting in an enlarged thyroid gland (goiter) or an overproduction of thyroid-stimulating hormone (TSH) by the pituitary gland, caused by a pituitary tumor.

30.12 What is a simple goiter?

A lack of iodine in the patient's diet (endemic, simple goiter) causes the thyroid gland to become enlarged.

30.13 Why is a simple goiter not common today?

This is seen less today because iodine is added to table salt.

30.14 What is hypopituitarism?

Hypopituitarism results when the pituitary gland is unable to secrete a normal amount of pituitary hormones.

30.15 What is hyperpituitarism?

The pituitary gland produces an excessive amount of growth hormone.

30.16 What is gigantism?

If hyperpituitarism occurs before epiphyseal closure, the patient (infants and children) has gigantism, resulting in an overgrowth of all body tissues.

30.17 What is acromegaly?

If hyperpituitarism occurs after epiphyseal closure, which is rare, the patient has acromegaly, resulting in bone thickening, growth in width (transverse growth), and enlarged organs (visceromegaly).

30.18 What is hyperprolactinemia?

This is an overproduction of the prolactin hormone that promotes lactation.

30.19 What is a common cause of hyperprolactinemia?

Excessive secretion is usually caused by a pituitary tumor (prolactinoma) and may also be caused by hypothyroidism, chronic kidney disease, and medications that affect the pituitary gland.

30.20 What is diabetes insipidus?

Either a decrease in antidiuretic hormone (ADH) production by the hypothalamus or the increased ADH by the pituitary gland causes a decreased ability of the kidneys to concentrate urine. This results in the excretion of large amounts of diluted urine. The patient then drinks large amounts of fluid to replace the increased urine output.

30.21 What is metabolic syndrome?

These patients have a collection of symptoms that include high blood glucose, obesity, high blood pressure, and high triglycerides based on family history. Beta cells in the pancreas are unable to produce sufficient insulin, whereas the liver produces a higher level of glucose. The patient is also insulin resistant. This syndrome leads to cardiovascular disease.

30.22 What is the syndrome of inappropriate secretion of antidiuretic hormone (SIADH)?

SIADH is caused by too much ADH being secreted by the posterior pituitary gland. ADH is responsible for controlling the amount of water reabsorbed by the kidney; it prevents the loss of too much fluid. When too much water is detected, ADH production or secretion is halted.

30.23 What is Addison's disease?

Addison's disease is inadequate secretion of corticosteroids from the adrenal cortex, resulting from damage to the adrenal cortex.

30.24 What is Cushing's syndrome?

The adrenal cortex secretes an excess of glucocorticoids or the pituitary gland an excess of adrenocorticotropic hormone (ACTH) as a result of a pituitary tumor, adrenal tumor, or from ongoing glucocorticoid therapy.

30.25 What is Conn's syndrome?

Conn's syndrome (primary aldosteronism) occurs when the adrenal cortex is secreting an excessive amount of aldosterone caused by an adrenal tumor, a malfunctioning adrenal cortex, or sources outside the adrenal gland producing aldosterone.

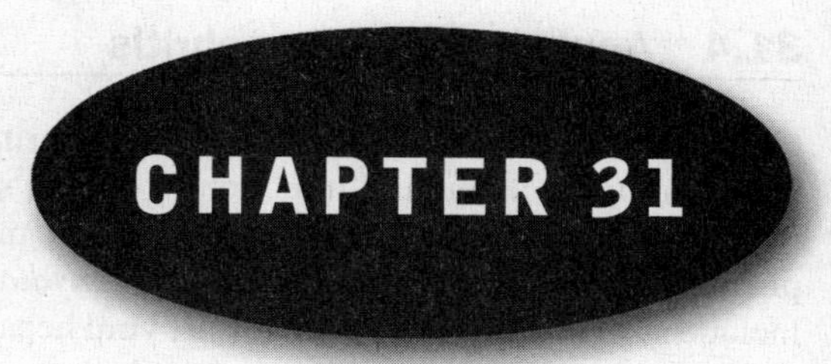

The Genitourinary System

31.1 Definition

The genitourinary system refers to the parts of the body involved in the production and transport of urine, as well as the surrounding structures.

The kidneys are found in the posterior part of the upper abdominal area, relatively protected by the lower ribs. They are lateral to the spinal column. The left kidney is higher than the right kidney because of the location of the liver within the abdomen. The renal artery supplies blood to the kidneys. The nephron is the functional unit of the kidney, the area in which urine is formed. Within the nephron, there is a long tubule. This initially surrounds the glomerulus in an area called Bowman's capsule.

Bowman's capsule narrows into a proximal convoluted tubule that has many curves and eventually straightens into a downward loop of Henle, which makes a sharp turn to come back up into the cortex of the kidney. The initial upward portion of the loop of Henle is thin and then becomes thick, which is the distal convoluted tubule.

The kidneys are responsible for filtering wastes from the bloodstream; they aid in the control of fluid and electrolyte balance, acid-base balance, blood pressure control through production of renin, and red blood cell production through the production of erythropoietin.

As urine is produced within the kidneys, it travels through the ducts (ureters) to the bladder. Once the body senses the urge to empty the bladder, the detrusor muscles contract and the sphincter at the bladder neck relaxes to aid in emptying the urine.

The urine passes through the urethra to the outside. Male patients have a prostate gland located under the bladder, surrounding the urethra. Prostatic fluid is secreted from the gland into the urethra.

31.2 Benign Prostatic Hyperplasia (BPH)

The prostate gland is found just below the bladder in men, surrounding the urethra. As men age, the prostate enlarges, putting pressure on the surrounding structures and causing symptoms such as frequent urination and urinary retention. The enlargement of the prostate causes narrowing of the urethra and upward pressure on the lower border of the bladder. Urinary retention may develop, as the body has a harder time emptying the bladder. Hydronephrosis and dilation of the renal pelvis and ureter are complications of the urinary retention due to overgrowth of the prostate.

31.3 Bladder Cancer

Bladder cancer is typically a nonaggressive cancer that occurs in the transitional cell layer of the bladder. It is recurrent in nature. Less frequently, bladder cancer is found invading deeper layers of the bladder tissue. In these cases the cancer tends to be more aggressive. Exposure to industrial chemicals (paints, textiles), history of cyclophosphamide use, and smoking increase the risks for bladder cancer.

31.4 Acute Glomerulonephritis

Glomerulonephritis, also known as acute nephritic syndrome, is infection of the glomerulus and is typically preceded by an ascending infection or occurs secondary to another systemic disorder. Infectious causes include group A beta-hemolytic *streptococcus*, measles, mumps, cytomegalovirus, varicella, coxsackievirus, pneumonia caused by mycoplasma, *Chlamydia psittaci*, or pneumococcal infection. Systemic disorders include systemic lupus erythematosus, viral hepatitis B or C, thrombotic thrombocytopenia purpura, or multiple myeloma.

31.5 Kidney Cancer

Kidney cancer occurs when cancer cells create a tumor within the kidney. Exposure to chemicals, lead, and smoking all increase the risk of developing kidney cancer.

31.6 Kidney Stones

Kidney stones, also known as renal calculi or nephrolithiasis, occur within the kidneys. Stones can also form elsewhere within the urinary tract. The patient may not have any symptoms from kidney stones until the stone attempts to move down the ureter toward the bladder.

Patients develop crystals within the urine. A slow flow of urine gives the crystals time to form a stone. Crystals may be formed from calcium, uric acid, cystine, or struvite. Medications such as diuretics can increase the risk of kidney stone formation in some patients at risk.

31.7 Prostate Cancer

Cancer of the prostate typically is found in the peripheral area of the prostate gland. Nodules may be palpable on digital rectal exam. There is a greater incidence as men age. African American males and those with a family history of the disease have a higher risk for prostate cancer. The symptoms of prostate cancer are the same as those of benign prostatic hypertrophy.

31.8 Pyelonephritis

Pyelonephritis is an infection involving the kidneys. Inflammation of the tissue accompanies the infectious process. The most common bacteria are *Escherichia coli, Klebsiella, Enterobacter, Proteus, Pseudomonas,* and *Staphylococcus saprophyticus.* Typically the infection begins in the lower urinary tract and ascends upward. Identification of infections and initiation of treatment are important to prevent the infection from getting worse.

31.9 Renal Failure

A decrease in renal function can occur in an acute (sudden) or chronic (progressive) manner. Acute renal failure can be broken down into prerenal, renal, and postrenal.

- **Prerenal Failure:** This is caused from diminished renal perfusion. Hypovolemia due to blood or fluid losses, diuretic use, third-spacing of fluids, reduced renal perfusion due to nonsteroidal anti-inflammatory drug (NSAID) use or congestive heart failure (CHF) can cause prerenal failure.

- **Renal Failure:** In acute care patients, this most commonly results from acute tubular necrosis. Drug-related reactions, particularly to antibiotics, may cause an allergic interstitial nephritis. Pyelonephritis or glomerulonephritis may also cause renal failure.
- **Postrenal Failure:** This is caused by some type of urinary tract obstruction, bladder outlet obstruction, a stone, prostate hypertrophy, or compression of ureter resulting from abdominal mass.

Chronic renal failure is an irreversible renal disease because of damaging effects on the kidneys caused by diabetes mellitus, hypertension, glomerulonephritis, HIV infection, polycystic kidney disease, or ischemic nephropathy.

31.10 Testicular Cancer

Cancer involving the testicle typically occurs in males in their teens or twenties. The cancer is hormonally dependent and tends to metastasize fairly quickly to lungs or bone. A painless nodule may be found by the patient. There is an increased incidence in patients with a history of cryptorchism.

31.11 Urinary Tract Infection (UTI)

Urinary tract infection (UTI) occurs when an infecting organism, typically gram-negative bacteria such as *E. coli,* enters the urinary tract. Inflammation of the local area occurs, followed by infection as the organism reproduces.

Often the bacteria are present on the skin in the genital area and enter the urinary tract through the urethral opening. The organism can also be introduced during sexual contact. The infection occurs as an uncomplicated, community-acquired infection in this setting.

Patients with a urinary catheter in place may also develop an infection because of the presence of the catheter, which allows a pathway for the bacteria to enter the bladder.

Instrumentation of the urinary tract (e.g., cystoscopy), also allows a pathway for bacteria to enter the bladder. Some of the instruments are not completely sterilized between patients; they are treated with a high-level disinfectant because of fiberoptics and lenses within because they would not withstand the high temperatures needed to sterilize. These infections would be considered nosocomial.

Solved Problems

Genitourinary System

31.1 What is a nephron?

A nephron is the functional unit of the kidney, the area in which urine is formed.

31.2 What is Bowman's capsule?

Within the nephron, there is a long tubule. This initially surrounds the glomerulus in an area called Bowman's capsule.

31.3 What are ureters?

As urine is produced within the kidneys, it travels through the ducts (ureters) to the bladder.

31.4 What are detrusor muscles?

Once the body senses the urge to empty the bladder, the detrusor muscles contract and the sphincter at the bladder neck relaxes to aid in emptying the urine.

31.5 What is benign prostatic hypertrophy (BPH)?

BPH is enlargement of the prostate.

31.6 What is bladder cancer?

Bladder cancer is typically a nonaggressive cancer that occurs in the transitional cell layer of the bladder.

31.7 What increases the risk of bladder cancer?

Exposure to industrial chemicals (paints, textiles), history of cyclophosphamide use, and smoking increase the risks for bladder cancer

31.8 What increases the risk of kidney cancer?

Kidney cancer occurs when cancer cells create a tumor within the kidney. Exposure to chemicals, lead, and smoking all increase the risk of developing kidney cancer.

31.9 What is acute glomerulonephritis?

Glomerulonephritis, also known as acute nephritic syndrome, is infection of the glomerulus and is typically preceded by an ascending infection or occurs secondary to another systemic disorder.

31.10 What are kidney stones?

Patients develop crystals within the urine. A slow flow of urine gives the crystals time to form a stone.

31.11 What medication increases the risk of kidney stone formation?

Diuretics increase the risk of kidney stone formation.

31.12 What is prostate cancer?

Cancer of the prostate typically is found in the peripheral area of the prostate gland. Nodules may be palpable on a digital rectal exam. The symptoms of prostate cancer are the same as those of BPH.

31.13 What is pyelonephritis?

Pyelonephritis is an infection involving the kidneys.

31.14 How does pyelonephritis develop?

Typically the infection begins in the lower urinary tract and ascends upward.

31.15 What is renal failure?

A decrease in renal function can occur in an acute (sudden) or a chronic (progressive) manner.

31.16 What is prerenal renal failure?

Prerenal renal failure is caused by diminished renal perfusion. Hypovolemia due to blood or fluid losses, diuretic use, third-spacing of fluids, reduced renal perfusion caused by NSAID use or congestive heart failure (CHF) can cause prerenal failure.

31.17 What is hypovolemia?

Hypovolemia is decreased fluid volume.

31.18 What is postrenal failure?

Postrenal failure is caused by some type of urinary tract obstruction, bladder outlet obstruction, a stone, prostate hypertrophy, or compression of ureter resulting from abdominal mass.

31.19 What is chronic renal failure?

Chronic renal failure is an irreversible renal disease due to damaging effects on the kidneys caused by diabetes mellitus, hypertension, glomerulonephritis, HIV infection, polycystic kidney disease, or ischemic nephropathy.

31.20 What is a urinary tract infection (UTI)?

A UTI occurs when an infecting organism, typically gram-negative bacteria such as *E. coli,* enters the urinary tract. Inflammation of the local area occurs, followed by infection as the organism reproduces.

31.21 What is a common cause of UTI?

Often the bacteria are present on the skin in the genital area and enter the urinary tract through the urethral opening.

31.22 Why is a patient with a urinary catheter at risk for a UTI?

Patients with a urinary catheter in place may also develop an infection because of the presence of the catheter which allows a pathway for the bacteria to enter the bladder.

31.23 How is nosocomial infection acquired?

Nosocomial infection is caused as a result of being hospitalized.

31.24 What causes hypovolemia?

Hypovolemia resulting from blood or fluid losses, diuretic use, third-spacing of fluids, reduced renal perfusion owing to NSAID use or congestive heart failure (CHF) can cause prerenal failure.

31.25 What is tubular necrosis?

Tubular necrosis is the death of tissues in the tubular portion of the kidney.

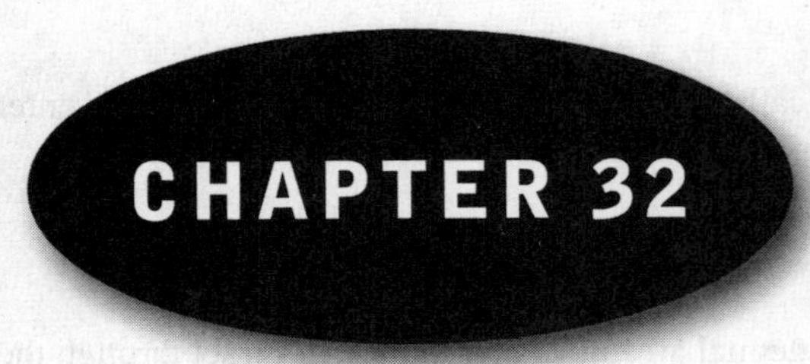

The Integumentary System

32.1 Definition

The outside covering of the body, or the skin, serves three major purposes. It prevents dehydration, regulates body temperature, and is the major deterrent of infection in the body. When this barrier is broken, whether by surgical incision, wound, cut, or scrape, the primary defense is no longer intact.

Superficial breaks in the skin may be treated on an outpatient basis. However, deeper wounds, and those involving the face and neck, may need more intense care with IV antibiotics. Skin is composed of several layers and is waterproof. Many skin manifestations are described using common terms.

Macules are small, flat-topped lesions, <1 cm in diameter, similar to a freckle. Papules are elevated lesions, also <1 cm in diameter. A wheal is a raised area filled with fluid and usually temporary, such as in hives.

A vesicle is a fluid-filled blister, often seen in shingles. Bullae are >1 cm in diameter and are fluid-filled blisters. A plaque is >1 cm in diameter, raised, and shallow.

A nodule is a solid lesion, up to 1 cm in diameter with depth. A tumor is >1 cm in diameter, and is solid with depth. A pustule is an elevation containing purulent material. Petechiae are <1 cm in diameter and are usually round areas of deposits of blood. A purpura is a large petechia.

32.2 Burns

Burns are damage to the skin and body tissues caused by flames, heat, cold, friction, radiation (sunburn), chemicals, or electricity. Burns are generally divided into three categories, depending on the damage.

A first-degree burn occurs with injury to the outer layer of skin called the epidermis. It is red and painful with some swelling.

A second-degree burn occurs when the epidermis is burned, as well as the next layer, the dermis. Severe pain, white and reddened areas, swelling, blisters, and perhaps drainage are seen.

A third-degree burn goes through all the layers of the skin and could involve underlying tissues. It is often painless because of destruction of the nerves in the area. The area looks black (termed eschar) and/or reddened.

Many drugs may make the skin more sensitive to the sun, producing the effect of sunburn with little exposure. Common medications with this effect include: amiodarone, carbamazepine, furosemide, naproxen, oral contraceptives, piroxicam, quinidine, quinolones, sulfonamides, sulfonylureas, tetracyclines, and thiazides, among others.

32.3 Dermatitis

Dermatitis is inflammation of the skin as a result of contact with an irritating substance such as a chemical, foreign substance, medication, or contact with a plant such as poison ivy. The skin may become reddened, irritated, and itchy.

The usual causes are allergic reactions. Often the patient has a history or a family history of asthma, allergy, or eczema. Some later symptoms may be the result of scratching of the skin. Often the cause may be a drug reaction, the body's immune system reacting to a medication.

32.4 Skin Cancers

Cancer of the skin is the most common type of cancer. The incidence of skin cancer is one of the fastest growing. Early detection is of the utmost importance because a cure is obtainable in the early stages.

Heredity may also be a factor. Skin cancer is usually divided into three major subtypes:

1. **Basal Cell:** Most common
2. **Squamous Cell:** Second most common
3. **Melanoma:** Most fearsome

Basal cell carcinomas are directly related to sun damage, with most lesions occurring in sun-exposed areas. This type recurs frequently. Squamous cell carcinomas are often caused by sun exposure, may be difficult to distinguish from some changes in the skin, and spread more readily. Melanoma is the most deadly form of skin cancer; it usually occurs on the face or upper back. A mnemonic to aid in remembering melanoma characteristics may be helpful:

A—asymmetric shape
B—borders that are irregular
C—change in color
D—diameter larger than a pencil eraser
E—ever changing

32.5 Cellulitis

Cellulitis is an infection of the skin, caused by bacteria that enter the skin through an opening. The legs are the most common site of cellulitis, although it may occur anywhere that bacteria enter. The most common bacteria are *Streptococcus* and *Staphylococcus*.

Bacteria may enter through fissures in the feet from fungal infections, through cracks in dry skin, from insect bites, or cuts from shaving. The elderly, immunocompromised patients, and patients with lymphedema, diabetes, or poor circulation are at greatest risk.

32.6 Pressure Ulcers

A pressure ulcer starts on the skin and often progresses to deeper tissue; it is caused by impaired circulation to the tissue from pressure over a period of time. Without adequate blood flow and the nutrition it brings, the tissue die. Those often affected are confined to a wheelchair or bed, and unable to move themselves, not reducing the pressure frequently enough. It can take as little as a few hours in one position for a stage 1 pressure ulcer to develop. The usual sites of pressure ulcers, or bedsores, are on bony prominences, such as the buttocks, sacrum, heels, knees, and hips.

Friction from linens can impair the integrity of the skin, as can the shear force, when the skin moves in one direction and the deeper structures do not move. Assessment tools are available to predict the risk of pressure ulcers developing. A commonly used scale is the Braden scale, which includes such criteria as friction, the nutritional status of the patient, mobility and activity levels, moisture exposure of the skin, and any limitations of sensory perception.

32.7 Wounds and Healing

A wound is any break in the skin. It may be intentional, as with surgery, or unintentional, as a result of trauma. Types of wounds include surgical, penetrating (such as a knife), crushing, burn, lacerations, bites (human, animal), ulcers, and pressure ulcers. Immediately after a wound occurs, inflammation occurs with platelet aggregation. Next, leukocytes travel to the area for infection surveillance.

A proliferative phase starts when the epidermal cells move toward the wound, and cover the approximated wound edges, usually by the third day. The fibroblastic phase occurs with collagen and fibroblasts forming a scar. Wound healing occurs in various ways. Primary intention happens when edges are closely approximated and new tissue, or granulation, knits the close edges together.

Wound healing by secondary intention occurs in a larger wound in which the edges are farther apart. This is often intentional when the wound is infected, dirty, or from a bite. The granulation tissue builds across the surface of the wound forming a large clot and sequentially, a larger scar.

Solved Problems

Integumentary System

32.1 What is the purpose of skin?

The outside covering of the body, or the skin, serves three major purposes. It prevents dehydration, regulates body temperature, and is the major deterrent of infection in the body.

32.2 What are macules?

Macules are small, flat-topped lesions, <1 cm in diameter, similar to a freckle.

32.3 What are papules?

Papules are elevated lesions, also <1 cm in diameter.

32.4 What is a wheal?

A wheal is a raised area filled with fluid and is usually temporary, such as in hives.

32.5 What is a vesicle?

A vesicle is a fluid-filled blister, often seen in shingles.

32.6 What are bullae?

Bullae are >1 cm in diameter and are fluid-filled blisters.

32.7 What is plaque?

A plaque is >1 cm in diameter, raised, and shallow.

32.8 What is a nodule?

A nodule is a solid lesion, up to 1 cm in diameter with depth.

32.9 What is a pustule?

A pustule is an elevation containing purulent material.

32.10 What are petechiae?

Petechiae are <1 cm in diameter and are usually round areas of deposits of blood.

32.11 What is a purpura?

A purpura is a large petechia.

32.12 What are burns?

Burns are damage to the skin and body tissues caused by flames, heat, cold, friction, radiation (sunburn), chemicals, or electricity. Burns are generally divided into three categories, depending on the damage.

32.13 What is a second-degree burn?

A second-degree burn occurs when the epidermis is burned, as well as the next layer, the dermis. Severe pain, white and reddened areas, swelling, blisters, and perhaps drainage are seen.

32.14 What is a third-degree burn?

A third-degree burn goes through all the layers of the skin and could involve underlying tissues. It is often painless because of destruction of the nerves in the area.

32.15 What is eschar?

Eschar is the area of burned skin in a third-degree burn that looks black.

32.16 What causes basal cell carcinomas?

Basal cell carcinomas are directly related to sun damage, with most lesions occurring in sun-exposed areas.

32.17 What are squamous cell carcinomas?

Squamous cell carcinomas are often caused by sun exposure, may be difficult to distinguish from some changes in the skin, and spread more readily.

32.18 What is melanoma?

Melanoma is the most deadly form of skin cancer; it usually occurs on the face or upper back.

32.19 What are characteristics of a melanoma?

A—asymmetric shape

B—borders that are irregular

C—change in color

D—diameter larger than a pencil eraser

E—ever changing

32.20 What is cellulitis?

Cellulitis is an infection of the skin, caused by bacteria that enter the skin through an opening.

32.21 What causes a pressure ulcer?

A pressure ulcer starts on the skin and often progresses to deeper tissue; it is caused by impaired circulation to the tissue from pressure over a period of time. Without adequate blood flow and the nutrition it brings, the tissue will die.

32.22 What is the Braden scale?

The Braden scale is a commonly used scale that includes such criteria as friction, the nutritional status of the patient, mobility and activity levels, moisture exposure of the skin, and any limitations of sensory perception.

32.23 What is a wound?

A wound is any break in the skin.

32.24 What is the proliferative phase of wound healing?

The proliferative phase starts when the epidermal cells move toward the wound, and cover the approximated wound edges, usually by the third day.

32.25 What is the fibroblastic phase of wound healing?

The fibroblastic phase occurs with collagen and fibroblasts forming a scar.

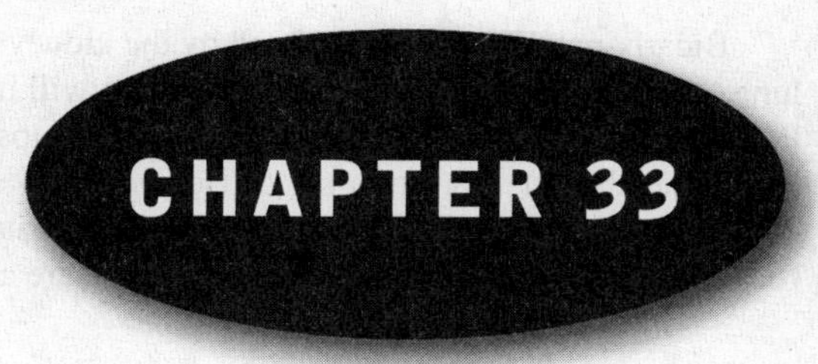

Fluids and Electrolytes

33.1 Definition

Fluids in the body are found in three basic places: within the cells (intracellular), outside the cells (extracellular), and within the tissue spaces (interstitial space or third space). A balance should be maintained to keep concentrations of both fluids and electrolytes in the proper areas for normal function.

The cell walls are semipermeable to allow for movement (diffusion) of molecules. This helps to maintain osmotic pressure. Edema occurs when too much fluid enters the interstitial space. Peripheral edema usually collects in subcutaneous areas. The higher hydrostatic pressure in the vessel causes fluids to move into the interstitial areas that have lower pressure, allowing the fluid to build up.

Normal osmolarity of plasma is 270 to 300 mOsm/L. Isotonic or normotonic fluids have similar concentrations. This prevents fluids from shifting into spaces they do not belong. Hypertonic solutions have a concentration >300 mOsm/L and exert greater pressure, which pulls water from the isotonic area to the hypertonic solution in an attempt to equalize the osmolarity. Hypotonic solutions have a concentration of <270 mOsm/L and exert less pressure, which allows water to be pulled from the hypotonic area into the isotonic area.

33.2 Hormonal Regulation of Fluids and Electrolytes

Aldosterone is secreted by the adrenal cortex in response to sodium changes. Where sodium goes, water follows. Aldosterone signals the tubules within the nephrons in the kidneys to reabsorb sodium and therefore water. This increases blood osmolarity. Aldosterone also aids in control of potassium levels.

Renin is secreted by the kidneys in response to changes in sodium or fluid volume. In the circulation, renin acts on a plasma protein called renin substrate (also called angiotensinogen), converting it to angiotensin I. In the pulmonary circulation, angiotensin-converting enzyme converts angiotensin I to angiotensin II. This causes vascular constriction and aldosterone secretion.

Antidiuretic hormone (ADH) is produced in the brain and stored in the posterior pituitary. It is released when there is a change in the osmolarity of the blood. ADH acts on the renal tubules, causing them to reabsorb more water, which decreases blood osmolarity. When the osmolarity gets too low, the release of ADH is not needed and water is excreted in the urine.

Natriuretic peptides are secreted in response to increases in blood volume and blood pressure. When atrial natriuretic peptide (ANP) and brain natriuretic peptide (BNP) are secreted, kidney reabsorption of sodium is inhibited and the glomerular filtration rate is increased. Blood osmolarity is decreased and urine output is increased.

33.3 Acid-Base Balance

Maintaining acid-base balance keeps the pH level within the normal range of 7.35 to 7.45. The lungs and kidneys are integral in maintaining the normal acid-base balance. The body constantly monitors the pH level and makes adjustments in an attempt to correct any abnormalities.

Bicarbonate (HCO_3) is regulated by the kidneys. Partial pressure of carbon dioxide (PCO_2) is regulated by the lungs. If the patient develops acidosis, there will be a low pH and either a drop in HCO_3 (metabolic) or a rise in PCO_2 (respiratory). If the patient develops alkalosis there will be an increase in pH and either an increase in HCO_3 (metabolic) or a drop in PCO_2 (respiratory).

In an attempt to maintain as normal an internal environment as possible, the body attempts to compensate for the changes that are occurring. The lungs are able to correct much more rapidly than the kidneys.

33.4 Hyponatremia

Hyponatremia is an abnormally low amount of sodium in the blood. Low levels of sodium may be caused by loss of sodium from the body, movement of sodium from the blood to other spaces, or dilution of sodium concentration within the plasma.

Some causes include excretion of sodium, water imbalance, hormonal imbalance (such as excess ADH), ecstasy (methylenedioxymethamphetamine) use, hypothyroidism, renal failure, diuretics, diarrhea, vomiting, and wound drainage.

33.5 Hypernatremia

Hypernatremia is an abnormally high amount of sodium in the blood. Fluid volume may be altered as a result of changes in the levels of sodium. A mild rise in sodium levels causes tissue that is normally excitable to become more irritable (e.g., cardiac muscle).

The osmolarity of extracellular fluid also increases as the sodium level increases. This is an attempt to correct the sodium increase by bringing more fluid from the cells into the extracellular area. These dehydrated, more irritable cells have a decreased ability to respond to stimuli.

Causes may include insufficient water intake (patients who are NPO), insufficient sodium excretion because of hormone imbalance, renal failure, corticosteroids, increased sodium intake or increased water loss because of fever, hyperventilation, increased metabolism, and dehydration because of sweating, vomiting, or diarrhea.

33.6 Hypocalcemia

Hypocalcemia is an abnormally low level of calcium in the blood. Decreased levels of calcium may be caused by inadequate intake or absorption (vitamin D deficiency, malabsorption), excess loss (associated with burns, renal disease, diuretics, or alcoholism), endocrine disorders (e.g., hypoparathyroidism), decreased serum albumin, hyperphosphatemia, or sepsis.

33.7 Hypercalcemia

Hypercalcemia is an abnormally high amount of calcium in the blood. Excess intake of calcium such as supplements or antacids or altered excretion of calcium as in patients with renal failure or those taking thiazide diuretics may cause hypercalcemia. Patients may also develop elevated calcium levels with prolonged immobility, glucocorticoid use, hyperthyroidism, hyperparathyroidism, lithium use, dehydration, or malignancies with metastasis to the bone.

33.8 Hypokalemia

Hypokalemia is a lower-than-normal level of potassium in the blood. A balance between the amount of potassium within the cell (intracellular) and outside the cell (extracellular) is necessary. This allows the resting potential of the cell membrane to be maintained. When there are low potassium levels, a greater-than-normal stimulus is needed to depolarize the cell membrane.

Many cells become more sluggish, especially nerve cells. However, cardiac cells become more excitable. Fluid losses caused by diuretics or diarrhea, endocrine disorders such as hyperthyroidism or hyperaldosteronism, insufficient intake of potassium, and low magnesium levels can all contribute to low potassium levels. Dietary intake is the main source of potassium, so patients with poor nutritional intake or prolonged NPO status are also at risk for hypokalemia.

33.9 Hyperkalemia

Hyperkalemia is an elevated level of potassium in the blood. Dietary intake is the main source of potassium. Patients are at risk for hyperkalemia when there is excessive ingestion of potassium-rich foods or salt substitutes, they are on medications that cause potassium retention (ACE inhibitors, angiotensin receptor blockers, potassium-sparing diuretics such as amiloride or spironolactone, NSAIDs, trimethoprim, pentamidine), or there is excess release of potassium from the cells (hemolysis, acidosis, low insulin levels, beta blocker use, digoxin overdose, succinylcholine, or rhabdomyolysis).

33.10 Hypomagnesemia

Hypomagnesemia is a lower-than-normal magnesium level in the blood. Low serum levels of magnesium can be caused by lack of sufficient intake or absorption (malnutrition, vomiting, diarrhea, celiac disease, Crohn's disease), excess excretion of magnesium (renal loss, chronic alcohol intake, diuretic use, aminoglycoside antibiotics, antineoplastics), or intracellular movement of magnesium (ascites, hyperglycemia, insulin administration). The cell membranes become more excitable in the setting of low magnesium levels. Patients may also have associated imbalances of potassium and calcium.

33.11 Hypermagnesemia

Hypermagnesemia is a greater-than-normal amount of magnesium in the blood. Patients with poor renal function or long-term abuse of magnesium-containing compounds have difficulty excreting magnesium.

The excess of magnesium in the blood causes the cell membranes to become less excitable than normal, requiring greater stimuli than would normally be needed to cause a required effect. As the magnesium level continues to rise, the cell membrane becomes more resistant to its natural stimuli.

33.12 Metabolic Acidosis

The acid-base balance of the blood is thrown off, causing it to become more acidic. There is an arterial pH of <7.35. There may be an overproduction of hydrogen ions (lactic acidosis in fever or seizures, diabetic ketoacidosis, starvation, alcohol or aspirin intake), deficient elimination of hydrogen ions (renal failure), deficient production of bicarbonate ions (renal failure, pancreatic insufficiency), or excess elimination of bicarbonate ions (diarrhea).

33.13 Metabolic Alkalosis

The acid-base balance of the blood is basic because of either a decrease in acidity or an increase in bicarbonate. Alkalosis is often associated with decreased levels of potassium or calcium. Metabolic alkalosis may be caused by excess intake of antacids, blood transfusions, long-term parenteral nutrition, prolonged vomiting or nasogastric suctioning, Cushing's disease, use of thiazide diuretics, or excess aldosterone.

33.14 Hypophosphatemia

Hypophosphatemia is a lower-than-normal amount of phosphorus in the blood. Chronic alcohol use, chronic obstructive pulmonary disease, asthma medications (loop diuretics, corticosteroids, adrenergic agonists, xanthine derivatives) are associated with low phosphate levels. Vitamin D is important in the intestinal absorption of phosphate. Parathyroid hormone stimulates the release of phosphate from the bone tissue. An overproduction can lead to hypophosphatemia.

33.15 Hyperphosphatemia

Hyperphosphatemia is a higher-than-normal amount of phosphorus in the blood. Patients may develop increased phosphate levels as a result of renal insufficiency, increase in phosphorus intake (supplements, laxatives, enemas, excess vitamin D), hypoparathyroidism, rhabdomyolysis, or as a result of cell destruction from chemotherapy. As phosphate levels increase, calcium levels decrease.

33.16 Dehydration

Dehydration is a state of having less-than-normal body fluids, caused by an excess loss of fluids or an inadequate intake of fluids. Dehydration may be actual or relative. A relative dehydration exists when the amount of fluid and electrolytes in the body is correct, but the placement is not correct.

If fluid shifting has occurred and the fluid is now in the interstitial areas rather than in the circulating blood volume, the patient may actually be experiencing a relative dehydration. Even though there is adequate fluid within the body, it cannot be used at this time. More commonly, dehydration is actual and caused by loss of fluid from the body or lack of adequate hydration.

Solved Problems

Fluids and Electrolytes

33.1 What is the interstitial space?

The interstitial space is the fluid within the tissue spaces.

33.2 What is edema?

Edema occurs when too much fluid enters the interstitial space.

33.3 What is peripheral edema?

Peripheral edema usually collects in the subcutaneous layer of skin.

33.4 What is normal osmolarity of plasma?

Normal osmolarity of plasma is 270 to 300 mOsm/L. Isotonic or normotonic fluids have similar concentrations. This prevents fluids from shifting into spaces they do not belong.

33.5 What are hypertonic solutions?

Hypertonic solutions have a concentration >300 mOsm/L and exert greater pressure, which pulls water from the isotonic area to the hypertonic solution in an attempt to equalize the osmolarity.

33.6 What are hypotonic solutions?

Hypotonic solutions have a concentration of <270 mOsm/L and exert less pressure, which allows water to be pulled from the hypotonic area into the isotonic area.

33.7 What is aldosterone?

Aldosterone is secreted by the adrenal cortex in response to sodium changes. Where sodium goes, water follows. Aldosterone signals the tubules within the nephrons in the kidneys to reabsorb sodium and therefore water. This increases blood osmolarity. Aldosterone also aids in control of potassium levels.

33.8 What is renin?

Renin is secreted by the kidneys in response to changes in sodium or fluid volume. In the circulation, renin acts on a plasma protein called renin substrate (also called angiotensinogen), converting it to angiotensin I. In the pulmonary circulation, angiotensin-converting enzyme converts angiotensin I to angiotensin II. This causes vascular constriction and aldosterone secretion.

33.9 What is antidiuretic hormone (ADH)?

ADH is produced in the brain and stored in the posterior pituitary. It is released when there is a change in the osmolarity of the blood. ADH acts on the renal tubules, causing them to reabsorb more water, which decreases blood osmolarity. When the osmolarity gets too low, the release of ADH is not needed and water is excreted in the urine.

33.10 What are natriuretic peptides?

Natriuretic peptides are secreted in response to increases in blood volume and blood pressure. When atrial natriuretic peptide (ANP) and brain natriuretic peptide (BNP) are secreted, kidney reabsorption of sodium is inhibited and the glomerular filtration rate is increased. Blood osmolarity is decreased and urine output is increased.

33.11 What regulates bicarbonate?

The kidneys regulate bicarbonate (HCO_3).

33.12 What regulates partial pressure of carbon dioxide?

The lungs regulate partial pressure of carbon dioxide (PCO_2).

33.13 What is alkalosis?

If the patient develops alkalosis, there is an increase in pH and either an increase in HCO_3 (metabolic) or a drop in PCO_2 (respiratory).

33.14 What is hyponatremia?

Hyponatremia is an abnormally low amount of sodium in the blood.

33.15 What is hypernatremia?

Hypernatremia is an abnormally high amount of sodium in the blood.

33.16 What is hypocalcemia?

Hypocalcemia is an abnormally low level of calcium in the blood.

33.17 What is hypercalcemia?

Hypercalcemia is an abnormally high amount of calcium in the blood.

33.18 What is hypokalemia?

Hypokalemia is a lower-than-normal level of potassium in the blood.

33.19 What is hyperkalemia?

Hyperkalemia is an elevated level of potassium in the blood.

33.20 What is hypomagnesemia?

Hypomagnesemia is a lower-than-normal magnesium level in the blood.

33.21 What is hypermagnesemia?

Hypermagnesemia is a greater-than-normal amount of magnesium in the blood.

33.22 What is hypophosphatemia?

Hypophosphatemia is a lower-than-normal amount of phosphorus in the blood.

33.23 What is hyperphosphatemia?

Hyperphosphatemia is a higher-than-normal amount of phosphorus in the blood.

33.24 What is dehydration?

Dehydration is a state of having less-than-normal body fluids, because of an excess loss of fluids or an inadequate intake of fluids.

33.25 Why is an electronystagmongram administered?

An electronystagmongram is administered to assess the underlying cause of loss of balance and vertigo.

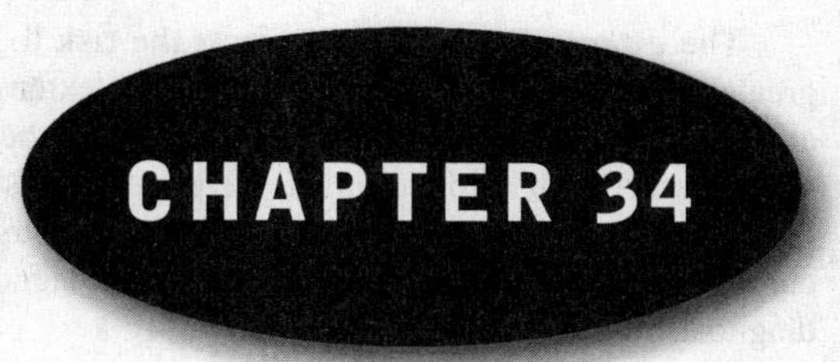

Perioperative Care

34.1 Definition

The care of the surgical patient ideally begins when the patient is first informed of the need for surgery. The surgical procedure may be a sudden, unexpected event for the patient, resulting in stress and anxiety (e.g., necessary surgery following trauma) or may be something that the patient has planned (e.g., a liposuction) far in advance.

The more time the patient has to prepare for surgery, both physically and emotionally, the better able the patient is to cope with the physiological stresses of the surgery. Nurses and other allied health professionals are in a position to care for the patient, provide necessary education, act as patient advocate, and encourage health promotion behaviors.

34.2 Surgical Classifications

The American Society of Anesthesiology categorizes surgical procedures based on the degree of risk to the patient. The urgency, location, extent, and reason for the procedure are all considered, as well as the patient's age; preexisting cardiovascular, respiratory, and neurologic statuses; endocrine disorders; malignancies; nutritional, fluid, and electrolyte status; abnormal laboratory findings; abnormal vital signs; and presence of infection. The risks of doing the surgery are weighed against the risks of not doing the surgery.

There are some cases in which the risk of surgery is very high, but the patient may certainly die if the surgery is not performed (patients with uncontrolled internal bleeding following a gunshot or stabbing, for example).

The anatomical *location* of the surgery affects the degree of risk to the patient. Surgical procedures performed within the thoracic cavity or skull are a greater risk to the patient than procedures performed on the extremities. Surgical procedures involving vital organs such as the heart, lungs, or brain carry a higher risk. The procedures that involve a greater potential for blood loss such as vascular surgery, also involve greater risk.

The degree of *urgency* of the procedure is described as emergent, urgent, or elective. Emergent procedures need to be performed immediately after identifying the need for surgery. Examples include surgery to stop bleeding from trauma, shooting, or stabbing, or dissection of an aortic aneurysm. Urgent procedures are scheduled after the determination of surgical need is made. Examples include tumor removal and removal of kidney stones. Elective procedures are scheduled in advance at a time that is convenient for both patient and surgeon. Postponement of the surgery for several weeks or even months will not cause harm to the patient. Examples include joint replacement procedures and cosmetic procedures.

The *extent* of the surgery affects the risk to the patient. The more extensive the surgical procedure, the greater the potential risk to the patient. More extensive surgical procedures cause more physical insult to the body and typically require a longer duration of anesthesia. The anesthesia can also cause stress to the patient's system, interact with medications in the patient's system, and must be metabolized out of the body.

The *reason* for surgery is another way that surgical procedures are classified. The purpose may be diagnostic, curative, restorative, palliative, or cosmetic. Diagnostic procedures are performed to obtain a biopsy for definitive diagnosis of a mass.

Curative procedures are performed to remove a diseased area such as a lumpectomy for breast cancer or an appendectomy. Restorative procedures are performed to restore function such as joint replacements.

Palliative procedures are procedures performed primarily for comfort measures such as tumor debulking. Cosmetic procedures are typically performed at the patient's request; at times some cosmetic procedures may fall into restorative (repairing damage or a congenital defect), curative, or diagnostic (in the setting of skin cancer).

The perioperative period can be broken down into the *preoperative* (time before the surgery), *intraoperative* (time during the surgery), and the *postoperative* (time following the surgery until recovery) periods.

34.3 Preoperative Period

The preoperative period, the time before surgery, is used to prepare the patient for surgery both physically and psychologically. Ideally there is time to correct as many abnormalities as possible before the surgical procedure.

For patients having a scheduled procedure with a significant anticipated blood loss, this is the time to donate blood to be banked for use in their surgery and begin to take iron, folic acid, vitamin B_{12}, and vitamin C to aid in red blood cell production. Preoperative clearance is given, informed consent is obtained, and preoperative teaching occurs during this time.

34.4 Preoperative Clearance

This is where the patient's primary care provider states that the patient is medically able to undergo surgery. The patient's primary care provider typically gives preoperative clearance for surgery. This physician, nurse practitioner, or physician's assistant is familiar with the patient's medical history and current medications and is able to adequately assess the impending risk of the surgery to the patient.

Things to consider when providing clearance for the patient include the type of surgical intervention planned, the potential for blood loss during surgery, the patient's age, general health and comorbidities, past medical and surgical history, current medications, use of herbal remedies or supplements, alcohol use, smoking history, substance use, allergies, family history including problems with surgery, and diagnostic testing results.

Diagnostic studies often include a CBC (to identify anemia or signs of infection), a chemistry panel (to identify electrolyte imbalance, abnormal glucose, liver or renal function), a urinalysis (to identify infection, protein, glucose), PT/INR/PTT (to identify blood clotting disorders), an ECG (to identify abnormal cardiac rhythms or damage to the myocardium), chest X-ray (to identify pulmonary pathology or enlargement of cardiac silhouette), or pulmonary function testing (for patients with respiratory disorders such as asthma or emphysema).

CT scans, MRIs, or PET scans may be ordered for individual patients depending on their medical history, type of surgical procedure planned, and results of other diagnostic studies.

34.5 Informed Consent

An informed consent is written approval signed by the patient that is obtained before any invasive or dangerous procedure. The reason for the surgery, type and extent of surgery to be performed, risks of the procedure, the person to perform the procedure, alternative options and their associated risks, and risks associated with anesthesia are all explained to the patient.

It is the surgeon's responsibility to make sure this information is explained to the patient. The patient must be a competent adult for his or her signature to be valid. If the patient has been given medications that alter his or her ability to reason or make judgments, the consent is not valid. The nurse witnesses the patient's signature on the consent form.

34.6 Preoperative Teaching

Explaining normal preoperative routines to the patient can be very helpful, so the patient knows what to expect. The nurse needs to be familiar with the types of surgical procedures and what the expected postoperative course will entail. The extent of the procedure, type of incision, presence of any tubes or drains, and anticipated pain level after the surgery will help guide the type of teaching necessary for the patient.

Preoperatively the patient can expect to be NPO (nothing by mouth), or not allowed to eat or drink anything for several hours before the procedure. The time frame depends on the extent and location of procedure, the type of anesthesia, and the scheduled time of surgery. An exception to this NPO rule would be for patients who need to take oral medications the morning of surgery.

Cardiovascular, diabetic, and certain other medications may need to be taken even though the patient is not to eat or drink anything else. An intravenous access site is obtained before the surgery. Fluids can be administered to the patient in this way. The access also allows for giving the patient medications intravenously for rapid action. Fluids are routinely given in the operating room and the immediate recovery period. The patient may have continued intravenous fluids for more extensive procedures.

Skin preparation may only involve washing of the surgical site in the operating room with an antimicrobial solution. Other patients may need to have removal of hair from the surgical site. This may be with a razor or a depilatory agent. It is important not to cut the skin if you are shaving a surgical site; small cuts or abrasions on the skin allow for potential sites of infection. Depilatory agents can be caustic on the skin of some patients, causing irritation or a rash. A small spot test away from the surgical area is a good idea in a patient with known skin sensitivity or history of allergies.

For patients having planned surgery involving the intestinal tract, a bowel preparation is completed before the surgery. This is done to decrease the bacterial count within the intestinal tract. Cleansing of the bowel is also completed to empty the intestine of stool before the surgeon plans on cutting into either the small or large intestines. Both of these preparations help to reduce the possibility of infection in the postoperative period.

For patients who will have tubes or drains in place in the postoperative period, a simple explanation of what to expect can help to alleviate some anxiety. Availability of pain medication in the postoperative period should be explained to the patient. In many instances, the patient is able to manage his or her own pain medication.

For outpatient procedures, patients may be given a prescription for an oral pain medication before the procedure. This way the medication is available when the patient gets home from the surgery. For postoperative patients in the hospital, many patients have an intravenous patient-controlled analgesia (PCA) for pain management in which pain medication is delivered via a pump.

Typically a small basal dose of narcotic is delivered all the time. These patients also have the ability to press a button whenever they are experiencing pain. The pump monitors the amount and timing of each dose of pain medication. If the patient is due for medication, a dose is administered; if the patient is not due for medication, no dose is administered.

34.7 Transfer of the Patient

Most facilities have a preoperative checklist to assist the nurse to make sure that all the needed components have been checked before sending the patient to the operating room (OR). All pertinent documentation—the signed consent form, the patient's chart, and current lab results—accompanies the patient to the OR.

34.8 Intraoperative Period

Members of the surgical team include the surgeon, a surgical assistant, an anesthesiologist or anesthetist, a circulating nurse, a scrub nurse or surgical tech, and a holding area nurse. The *surgeon* is the doctor who performs the surgery.

The *surgical assistant* may be another surgeon, a surgical resident, an RN first assist, or a physician's assistant. The person providing anesthesia and monitoring the vital signs of the patient is either an *anesthesiologist* (a physician) or a certified registered nurse *anesthetist* (CRNA).

The *circulating nurse* is a registered nurse who acts as the patient advocate, obtains the necessary supplies for the procedure, makes sure diagnostic studies and blood products are available if necessary, prepares the operative table, positions the patient (padding bony prominences if necessary), and cleanses the skin in the operative area before positioning surgical drapes.

The *scrub nurse* or *surgical tech* sets up the sterile field, assists with draping the patient, and hands sterile supplies into the operative field and takes used instruments from the surgeon. The circulating nurse and scrub nurse (or surgical tech) together count all instruments, sponges, and sharps used in the surgical field. The count is performed before, during, and after the procedure.

The *holding area nurse* cares for the patients who have been brought into the operating room suite but who are not yet ready to go into the operating room. The holding area nurse may be managing several patients at one time and can also help to transport and transfer the patient.

Before entering the operating room, the members of the surgical team scrub at the sink just outside the room in which the surgery will be performed. Before starting the scrub, the team member applies a mask with face shield or goggles.

The surgical scrub is usually timed and covers the area from the fingertips to 2 inches above the elbows. The surgical scrub renders the skin clean, not sterile. After the scrub, the skin is dried with a sterile towel. A sterile gown, then sterile gloves are applied. The front of the gown is considered sterile in the front from two inches below the neck to the waist and from the elbow to the wrist. The circulating nurse puts on the gown and gloves unassisted, and then assists the other members of the team into their gown and gloves as they enter the room.

34.9 Risk for Injury

During the surgery, the patient is anesthetized and cannot tell you if there is pressure anywhere. The patient is positioned to allow for maximal access to the operative site. This sometimes causes unnatural positioning of the patient or the patient's extremities. The operative table is padded to decrease pressure on the patient.

There may be additional padding added to areas of flexion or bony prominences to reduce the risk of pressure ulcer formation or nerve damage because of positioning. Heat loss can occur during surgery.

The patient is sent to the operating room in a hospital gown, which may be pulled up or removed depending on the body location of the surgery. The body is draped for privacy so that only the surgical area is exposed. The temperature within the operating room is kept rather cool because the air exchange rate is higher within the operating room than in other rooms (to decrease bacterial counts), and the staff wear double layers of clothes. Warmers can be set up for the patients during certain procedures when heat loss is expected—a large, open operative site or a long duration of surgery.

At the end of the surgical procedure, the wound is closed. The closure is to hold the wound edges together and prevent contamination. Closure may be achieved with sutures (either absorbable or nonabsorbable), staples, or skin closure tape. Nonabsorbable sutures and staples have to be removed in the postoperative period.

Drains may be inserted near the operative site if significant wound drainage is anticipated. Some drains are attached to suction, some have self-suction, and some drain because of gravity. The wound site is covered with a sterile dressing before the patient is transferred out of the operating room.

34.10 Anesthesia

Anesthesia can be administered via general or regional routes (for major procedures) or conscious sedation (for minor procedures). General anesthesia renders the patient unconscious and incapable of breathing on his or her own; pain reception is also blocked. These patients must be intubated and mechanically ventilated for the duration of the anesthesia.

Regional anesthesia can be achieved through nerve blocks, or epidural or spinal anesthesia. Nerve blocks occur when an anesthetic agent is injected into an area immediately surrounding a particular nerve or nerve bundle. The nerve tissue becomes anesthetized, effectively causing the tissue that it supplies to become pain free.

With epidural anesthesia, an anesthetic agent is injected into the epidural space surrounding the spinal column, usually in the lower lumbar area.

The nerves become anesthetized as they leave the spinal column, causing the area of the body supplied by these nerves to become pain free. This anesthesia is most commonly associated with childbirth, but is used for many surgical procedures. Spinal anesthesia is not commonly used; the anesthetic agent is injected into the cerebrospinal fluid.

Patient positioning is very important, as gravity will cause the anesthetic agent to travel. The patient must remain flat after the procedure to prevent leakage of cerebrospinal fluid from the puncture site.

34.11 Postoperative Period

After the surgery, the patient enters the postoperative period. The immediate postoperative period requires close monitoring as the patient emerges from anesthesia. The patient is then transferred to either a same-day surgery area for discharge home that day or an inpatient surgical unit for care. After discharge from the hospital, the patient may need home care. Return to full activities may take several weeks.

34.12 Postanesthesia Care

The patient is transferred from the operating room to the postanesthesia care unit (PACU) for close monitoring in the immediate postoperative period. Initial assessment is focused on ABC: airway, breathing, and circulation.

The practitioner should monitor the patient's airway, gas exchange, pulse oximetry, oxygen delivery, accessory muscle use, and breath sounds. The patient can develop stridor because of edema or bronchospasm. The cardiovascular status is checked next. Vital signs are checked every 15 minutes until stabilized; pulse, blood pressure, and cardiac rhythm are monitored.

The surgical wound is checked for signs of drainage or bleeding. The dressing is checked. The drains are checked for output and patency. Tubes that need to be connected to suction (e.g., nasogastric tubes) are connected. Intravenous fluids are monitored. Neurologic assessment is performed to check level of consciousness.

Following general anesthesia, the patient follows a predictable progression in the return to consciousness. Initially there is muscular irritability, and then restlessness followed by pain recognition and the ability to reason and control behavior. Pupil responses are monitored, looking for bilaterally equal responses to light. Motor responses are monitored, looking initially for purposeful response to painful stimuli and later for response to command.

Pain management is begun during this time. As the anesthetic agent wears off, it is important to assess the patient's level of pain. This may be assessed through subjective information in patients who are conscious, or through more objective signs in patients who are still in semiconscious states.

Monitor for changes in vital signs [elevated pulse and blood pressure (BP)], changes in movement, and moaning. Expected pain levels can be estimated from the type of surgery and give a starting point for those patients as they begin to come out of the anesthesia. Gastrointestinal status is monitored for presence of nausea or vomiting. This may be a reaction or side effect to anesthesia. Check for abdominal distention and presence of bowel sounds.

Monitor drainage from the nasogastric tube; note the amount and color of drainage. Monitor laboratory results as indicated. Electrolyte levels, hemoglobin or hematocrit levels, blood urea nitrogen (BUN) and creatinine, arterial blood gases (ABGs), or other studies may be necessary in the immediate postoperative period. The necessary diagnostic studies depend on the patient's history, estimated blood loss during surgery, and type of procedure performed.

After the initial recovery time, the stable patient who is transferred from the PACU to the same-day surgical area continues to be monitored. Vital signs are taken, although not as frequently. Respiratory and cardiovascular functions are monitored. Cardiac rhythm is no longer monitored. The dressing is checked for any drainage. Bowel sounds are checked. Clear fluids are given if the patient is not experiencing nausea.

Patients are monitored for urinary output before being discharged to home. Patients who are admitted to the hospital are transferred from the PACU to a surgical unit. Vital signs, respiration, and cardiovascular status are checked. The dressing is monitored for drainage; drainage tubes are monitored for output. Intravenous lines are monitored for signs of infiltration and proper flow rates.

Bowel sounds are monitored. Patients who are unstable or who have had extensive procedures are transferred to intensive care for close monitoring. Nurses who are used to caring for complex, unstable patients care for these patients. Their vital signs are closely monitored. Some patients will still be on mechanical ventilation.

34.13 Postoperative Complications

The focus of care that is common for all postoperative patients is identification of complications. Common complications involve the cardiac, respiratory, and gastrointestinal areas, and infections.

34.14 Cardiovascular Complications

Patients may develop cardiovascular complications because of the physiologic stress of surgery, side effects of the anesthesia or other medications, or comorbidities. Myocardial infarction (MI), cardiac arrhythmias, or hypotension are likely during or in the immediate postoperative period.

When getting the patient out of bed for the first time after surgery, it is good practice to have the patient sit on the side of the bed for a minute or two before standing up to ascertain if the patient feels dizzy because of a drop in blood pressure associated with position change. Deep vein thrombosis (DVT) is a later vascular complication associated with inflammation and decreased mobility after surgery.

34.15 Respiratory Complications

Patients with preexisting respiratory disorders, obesity, thoracic or upper abdominal surgical procedures are at greater risk of developing respiratory complications postoperatively. After surgery, patients are not as mobile. This lack of physical activity leads to a diminished chest wall and diaphragmatic movement, resulting in a decreased amount of air exchange. Alveolar sacs can collapse, leading to areas of atelectasis. Pain medications can adversely affect respiratory status by decreasing respiratory drive.

Patients at increased risk for respiratory complications may develop pneumonia in the postoperative period because of diminished airflow, increased respiratory secretions, and inflammatory processes. Patients with increased risk for clotting or DVT, or those with hypercoagulable states are at risk for developing a pulmonary embolism.

34.16 Infection

The skin is the body's first line of defense against infection. During surgery this line of defense is penetrated. Even though the surgical procedure is performed in as aseptic an environment as possible, the possibility of infection still exists. Wound infections can develop in the postoperative period.

The wound may be contaminated before surgery such as with penetrating trauma, or may become infected during healing. The surface of the skin has bacteria that are naturally present, referred to as normal flora. These bacteria may enter the wound and cause infection. Nosocomial infections can also occur at the surgical site, caused by bacteria found elsewhere in the hospital. Infection within the surgical wound slow approximation of the wound edges, delaying wound healing.

34.17 Gastrointestinal Complications

Following administration of anesthesia or pain medication, patients may experience nausea, vomiting, constipation, or paralytic ileus. Nausea is a common side effect of both anesthesia and pain medications. A patient's reaction to anesthetic agents varies. Some patients have a lot of nausea after anesthesia that may last for several hours.

Abdominal surgery may cause direct visceral afferent stimulation, resulting in nausea and vomiting. Medications may act upon the chemoreceptor trigger zone, located within the medulla outside the blood–brain barrier. Once the patient begins vomiting, antiemetic medication may be necessary to break the cycle.

Opioid-based medications and decreased activity can cause both slowing of peristaltic activity, leading to constipation. Patients having abdominal procedures are at greater risk for paralytic ileus as a postoperative complication.

Solved Problems

Perioperative Care

34.1 What is an emergent procedure?

An emergent procedure must be performed immediately after identifying the need for surgery. Examples include surgery to stop bleeding from trauma, shooting, or stabbing, or dissection of an aortic aneurysm.

34.2 What is an urgent procedure?

An urgent procedure is scheduled after the determination of surgical need is made. Examples include tumor or kidney stone removal.

34.3 What is an elective procedure?

Elective procedures are scheduled in advance at a time that is convenient for both patient and surgeon. Postponement of the surgery for several weeks or even months will not cause harm to the patient. Examples include joint replacement procedures and cosmetic procedures.

34.4 What is the extent of the surgery?

The extent of the surgery affects the risk to the patient. The more extensive the surgical procedure, the greater the potential risk to the patient. More extensive surgical procedures cause more physical insult to the body and typically require a longer duration of anesthesia. The anesthesia can also cause stress to the patient's system, interact with medications in the patient's system, and must be metabolized out of the body.

34.5 What is a curative procedure?

A curative procedure is performed to remove a diseased area such as a lumpectomy for breast cancer or an appendectomy.

34.6 What is a palliative procedure?

Palliative procedures are procedures performed primarily for comfort measures such as tumor debulking.

34.7 What is a cosmetic procedure?

Cosmetic procedures are typically performed at the patient's request; at times some cosmetic procedures may fall into restorative (repairing damage or a congenital defect), curative, or diagnostic (in the setting of skin cancer).

34.8 What is the perioperative period?

The perioperative period is the time before surgery through the time following surgery when the patient is recovered.

34.9 What is the preoperative period?

The preoperative period is the time before surgery.

34.10 What is the intraoperative period?

The intraoperative period is the time during surgery.

34.11 What is the postoperative period?

The postoperative period is the time following surgery until recovery.

34.12 What occurs during the preoperative period?

The preoperative period, the time before surgery, is used to prepare the patient for surgery both physically and psychologically. Ideally there is time to correct as many abnormalities as possible before the surgical procedure.

34.13 What is preoperative clearance?

The patient's primary care provider states that the patient is medically able to undergo surgery.

34.14 What is purpose of the CBC test before surgery?

The CBC test is used to identify anemia and signs of infection before surgery.

34.15 What is the purpose of the PT/INR/PTT test before surgery?

The PT/INR/PTT test identifies blood clotting disorders.

34.16 What is an informed consent?

An informed consent is written approval signed by the patient that is obtained before any invasive or dangerous procedure. It explains the reason for the surgery, the type and extent of surgery to be performed, the risks of the procedure, the person to perform the procedure, alternative options and their associated risks, and the risks associated with anesthesia.

34.17 What is preoperative teaching?

The medical provider explains normal preoperative routines to the patient so the patient knows what to expect. Also explained are the extent of the procedure, type of incision, presence of any tubes or drains, and anticipated pain level after the surgery.

34.18 Who is a surgical assistant?

The surgical assistant may be another surgeon, a surgical resident, an RN first assist, or a physician's assistant.

34.19 What is a circulating nurse?

A circulating nurse is a registered nurse who acts as the patient advocate, obtains the necessary supplies for the procedure, makes sure diagnostic studies and blood products are available if necessary, prepares the operative table, positions the patient (padding bony prominences if necessary), and cleanses the skin in the operative area before positioning surgical drapes.

34.20 What might be a cause of nausea and vomiting following abdominal surgery?

Direct visceral afferent stimulation.

34.21 What is a scrub nurse or surgical tech?

The scrub nurse or surgical tech sets up the sterile field, assists with draping the patient, and hands sterile supplies into the operative field and takes used instruments from the surgeon. The circulating nurse and scrub nurse (or surgical tech) together count all instruments, sponges, and sharps used in the surgical field.

34.22 What is a holding area nurse?

The holding area nurse cares for patients who have been brought into the operating room suite but who are not yet ready to go into the operating room. The holding area nurse may be managing several patients at one time and can also help to transport and transfer the patient.

34.23 What is a surgical scrub?

The surgical scrub is usually timed and covers the area from the fingertips to 2 inches above the elbows. The surgical scrub renders the skin clean, not sterile.

34.24 What is general anesthesia?

General anesthesia renders the patient unconscious and incapable of breathing on his or her own; pain reception is also blocked. These patients must be intubated and mechanically ventilated for the duration of the anesthesia.

34.25 What is regional anesthesia?

Regional anesthesia can be achieved through nerve blocks, or epidural or spinal anesthesia. Nerve blocks occur when an anesthetic agent is injected into an area immediately surrounding a particular nerve or nerve bundle. The nerve tissue becomes anesthetized, effectively causing the tissue that it supplies to become pain free.

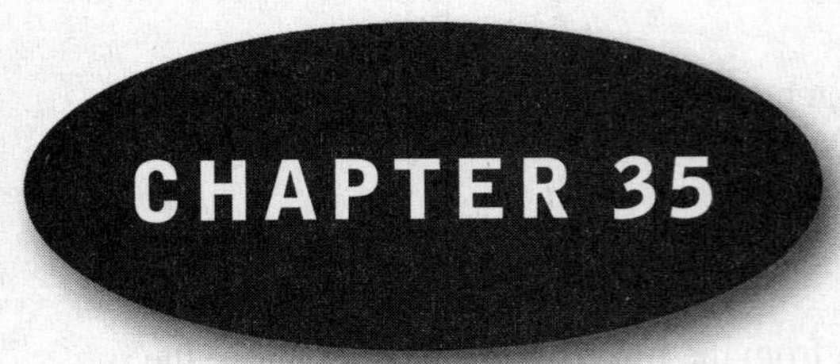

Women's Health

35.1 Definition

The menstrual cycle is the series of changes a woman's body goes through monthly to prepare for conception and a growing fetus. If fertilization does not occur, the uterus removes the prepared lining, termed menstrual bleeding. Menstruation begins in the early teens (menarche) and ends around age 50 (menopause). The average age of menarche for African Americans is 9 to 11 years, whereas for Caucasians it is 10 to 12 years.

The cycle is controlled by hormones from the hypothalamus, pituitary, ovaries, and the uterus. A normal menstrual cycle is 28 days, but only about 25% of women actually are on this schedule. The average can run from 21 to 35 days.

The menstrual cycle is often divided into three phases, dependent on the hormones. The beginning of menstruation is the start of the follicular phase, which lasts until day 14. As hormone levels are low, the thickened lining of the uterus begins to shed. The cramping that is felt is from small uterine contractions, helping to shed the lining.

An egg follicle begins to mature because of growing levels of follicle-stimulating hormone (FSH), which also causes estrogen secretion. The increase in estrogen causes the endometrium to mature and thicken. The last 5 days of the follicular phase plus the day of ovulation are the most fertile days. Upon the ovulation phase, on day 14, the oocyte, or egg, is released from the follicle because of a surge in luteinizing hormone (LH). The egg is expelled near the opening of one of the fallopian tubes (oviducts, uterine tubes), located laterally at the top of the uterus.

Fertilization usually occurs in one of the tubes. The embryo now travels to the uterus, the primary job of which is to sustain development. As it is a muscular organ, it is capable of great stretching. At the distal end of the uterus is the cervix that attaches to the superior portion of the vagina.

The luteal phase starts next with the LH causing the follicle to secrete progesterone instead of estrogen. Progesterone causes the endometrial lining to begin to thicken in preparation for implantation of a fertilized cell. Progesterone inhibits release of FSH and LH. If fertilization does not occur, the corpus luteum, containing the oocyte, dies, which lowers the level of progesterone. Sloughing of the lining begins about the twenty-eighth day of the cycle, resulting in a flow of blood and cellular debris through the vagina.

The cycle will begin again. Primary amenorrhea is the absence of menses by age 16. Secondary amenorrhea is the absence of menses for more than 6 months in a woman who previously was menstruating regularly.

35.2 Breast Cancer

Studies show that by age 80, about 1 in 8 women will have had breast cancer. Ten percent of all breast cancers are inherited. Two major genes have been identified—BRCA1 and BRCA2. Despite the research and advances in medicine, the cause of breast cancer is unknown. Some studies have implicated a higher fat diet. Some medications, like estrogen, seem to increase the risk of breast cancer. Exposure to radiation also increases the risk. Childlessness and delayed childbirth also may be factors.

35.3 Cervical Cancer

The Pap smear has markedly increased early detection of cervical cancer and thus decreased the mortality. Abnormal cells, cervical intraepithelial neoplasia (CIN), are the initial indication on a Pap smear, and are more common in women with HIV and those infected with human papillomavirus (HPV), subtypes 16, 18. Human papillomavirus more common in women with multiple sexual partners, those having sex at an early age, and those with HIV.

35.4 Dysmenorrhea

Menstrual pain occurring after ovulation for which no cause can be discerned is called dysmenorrhea. Dysmenorrhea is caused by the changing hormones in the reproductive cycle. Uterine contractions from prostaglandins and blood vessel constriction in the uterine lining cause the discomfort as the enriched lining prepares to be sloughed off.

35.5 Ectopic Pregnancy

Ectopic pregnancy occurs when the fertilized ovum implants in an area other than the uterus. Most ectopic pregnancies occur in the fallopian tubes; however, other possible sites for ectopic pregnancy include the ovary, cervix, and peritoneum. When the fertilized ovum is unable to get to the uterus, it may settle in the fallopian tube. Any blockage, stricture, previous surgery on the tube, infection, or inflammation may impede the ovum from its final, proper destination.

35.6 Endometrial Cancer

One of the most common gynecologic cancers in women, it is most often diagnosed in postmenopausal women. Abnormal tissue grows rapidly, affected most often by estrogen. Eventually, this abnormal tissue, hyperplasia, turns into a cancer. Some causes of elevated estrogen levels are exogenous estrogen, polycystic ovarian disease, and estrogen-producing tumors. Risk factors for endometrial cancer include endometrial hyperplasia, tamoxifen, type 2 diabetes, nulliparity, and obesity (estrogen is stored in adipose tissue).

35.7 Fibroids (Leiomyomas)

Leiomyomas are smooth muscle tumors of the uterus. Because they are hormone receptive, the tumors will change in size with the menses. It is unknown what causes the proliferation of these smooth muscle tumors. Fibroids are more common in African American women.

35.8 Infertility

Infertility is the inability of a reproductive-age couple to conceive after 12 months of unprotected sexual intercourse. More than 50% of the time the reproductive tract of the woman is at issue. Primary infertility is when a woman has never had a pregnancy; secondary is when it occurs in a woman who has had one or more pregnancies.

At fault may be decreased secretion of hormones from the anterior pituitary, failure to ovulate, endometriosis, or past infections causing blockage of the reproductive tract. Structural problems (blocked fallopian tubes, or anovulation), poor sperm motility and/or count, or multifactorial problems can cause infertility. Prior exposure to radiation, medications, exercise frequency, and menstrual cycle and length need to be evaluated.

35.9 Menopause

Menopause is defined as 12 months without a menses. Few follicles are left to mature, levels of hormones decline, ovulation no longer occurs, and the uterine lining no longer needs to thicken in preparation for a fertilized egg.

35.10 Ovarian Cancer

Ovarian cancer is the deadliest gynecologic cancer because it is usually advanced before it is detected. There is no proven screening test for ovarian cancer. There are no early signs. A woman who has never had a child or who has had only one or two children, is at higher risk for ovarian cancer. Women with a history of breast cancer, colon cancer, or a family history of these are at a higher risk of ovarian cancer. There is an association between endometriosis and ovarian cancer.

35.11 Benign Ovarian Masses

The most common ovarian cysts are follicular. The egg is enclosed in a follicle as it waits to be expelled monthly from the ovary. When the follicle does not open to allow the egg out or the follicle is not reabsorbed, a benign cyst, a fluid-filled sac, may result.

35.12 Pelvic Inflammatory Disease (PID)

Pelvic inflammatory disease (PID) is a variety of inflammation and infection of the upper genital tract, which includes the uterus, fallopian tubes, ovaries and other structures. It includes endometritis, salpingitis, oophoritis, tuboovarian abscess, and pelvic peritonitis. Bacteria from the cervix and vagina migrate to the upper genital tract.

Usual organisms include *Chlamydia trachomatis, Neisseria gonorrhoeae, Escherichia coli,* and *Bacteroides*. Most infections are caused by a mix of bacteria. PID occurs most often in sexually active women and is more common in adolescents. PID is more common with multiple sexual partners, a young age, unprotected sex, and a history of sexually transmitted disease.

35.13 Trophoblastic Disease

Trophoblastic neoplasias are abnormal cells growing from a shell that forms between the embryo and the endometrium. The four disease entities are called hydatidiform mole (partial or complete), invasive mole, choriocarcinoma, and placental site trophoblastic tumor. A complete mole is formed when an egg that has no DNA is fertilized by a sperm.

A partial mole has DNA from both parents and usually fetal parts. An invasive mole is a hydatidiform mole in the endometrium. Choriocarcinomas are tumors composed of trophoblasts with bleeding. Placental site trophoblastic tumors are trophoblasts that intrude the myometrium.

All are suggestive of malignancy and require a full metastatic workup, including CT scan of brain, kidneys, liver, and lung. There is thought to be a problem with the genetic material of the zygotes. The chances are increased with an older mother, prior molar pregnancy, and a history of miscarriage.

35.14 Pregnancy

Gestational age is measured from the first day of the last menstrual period (LMP). At each prenatal visit, the fundus (the top of the uterus) is measured as to its location in the abdomen. This information is used to assess the growth of the fetus. Pregnancy is usually divided into trimesters.

The *first trimester* is from 0 to 14 weeks, and starts at implantation. During this time, it is not uncommon to feel more fatigue, nausea, and morning sickness. At 2 months, the uterus is the size of a grapefruit. At 9 weeks, the embryo is called a fetus and is about 1 inch in length. During the first trimester, most major organs have developed.

The *second trimester* is from 14 to 28 weeks, and is characterized by less breast tenderness, less fatigue, and a diminishing of morning sickness. However, some back pain may begin, as well as stretch marks, heartburn, and hemorrhoids. At 16 weeks, the fundus is halfway between the pubic bone and the umbilicus. At 16 to 18 weeks, fetal movement may be felt. At 27 weeks, the fundus is 2 inches above the umbilicus.

The *third trimester* is from 28 weeks to birth. Less movement is felt because of the limited space for the fetus to move about. The mother may feel some respiratory difficulty as the uterus is directly underneath the diaphragm, pushing up the lungs. She may experience some edema, have difficulty sleeping, and an increased urge to urinate due to pressure on the bladder. She may feel mild abdominal cramping that is called Braxton-Hicks contractions.

35.15 Labor and Delivery

Labor is usually shorter in women who have previously had children than in first-time mothers. The average labor is anywhere from 12 to 24 hours. Labor is typically divided into three stages, with the first stage having two phases.

The first stage starts with the beginning of labor, which is uterine contractions that result in thinning (effacement) and dilation of the cervix. The first stage of labor ends with full dilation, at 10 cm, and complete effacement. This is the longest part of labor. Contractions are milder, last 60 to 90 seconds, and are 15 to 20 minutes apart in this first phase of labor, termed the latent phase.

The active phase occurs when the cervix dilates from 4 to 8 cm, contractions become stronger, last about 30 to 45 seconds, and are closer together. This is often when the membranes rupture, releasing amniotic fluid. A backache is common, as is some vaginal bleeding. When the cervix is fully dilated at 10 cm, the second stage of labor has started. This phase is fetal expulsion. Contractions continue, but feel different. There is pressure on the rectum, and a strong urge to push.

The second stage of labor ends with the birth of the baby. Delivery of the placenta, or afterbirth, is the third stage of labor. Contractions will continue, but are milder, as the uterus contracts, which helps to expel the placenta and slow the bleeding.

35.16 Postpartum

Postpartum is the time from birth to 6 weeks when involutionary changes occur.

35.17 Rh Incompatibility

Rh incompatibility is assessed on each mother during pregnancy. If the mother is Rh negative and the fetus is Rh positive, the mother may be exposed to the fetus's cells and develop antibodies to them.

35.18 Preeclampsia and Eclampsia

Preeclampsia is a condition that women may get in the latter half of pregnancy. It is pregnancy-induced hypertension and more often occurs in a first pregnancy. If preeclampsia is left untreated, eclampsia, which is seizures not related to a brain condition, will result.

The etiology of preeclampsia and eclampsia is unknown. Prepregnant hypertension, obesity, and poor nutrition may be contributing factors. First-time mothers have a greater risk of preeclampsia, as do women with a family history of the condition.

Solved Problems

Women's Health

35.1 What is the menstrual cycle?

The menstrual cycle is the series of changes a woman's body goes through monthly to prepare for conception and a growing fetus. If fertilization does not occur, the uterus will remove the prepared lining, termed menstrual bleeding. Menstruation begins in the early teens (menarche) and ends around age 50 (menopause). The average age of menarche for African Americans is 9 to 11 years, whereas for Caucasians it is 10 to 12 years.

35.2 What controls the menstrual cycle?

The cycle is controlled by hormones from the hypothalamus, pituitary, ovaries, and the uterus. A normal menstrual cycle is 28 days, but only about 25% of women actually are on this schedule. The average can run from 21 to 35 days.

35.3 What are the phases of the menstrual cycle?

The phases of the menstrual cycle are the follicular phase, ovulation phase, and the luteal phase.

35.4 What is the follicular phase?

The beginning of menstruation is the start of the follicular phase, which lasts until day 14. As hormone levels are low, the thickened lining of the uterus begins to shed. The cramping that is felt is from small uterine contractions, helping to shed the lining. An egg follicle begins to mature due to growing levels of follicle-stimulating hormone (FSH), which also causes estrogen secretion. The increase in estrogen causes the endometrium to mature and thicken.

35.5 What is the ovulation phase?

Upon the ovulation phase, on day 14, the oocyte, or egg, is released from the follicle due to a surge in luteinizing hormone (LH). The egg is expelled near the opening of one of the fallopian tubes, (oviducts, uterine tubes), located laterally at the top of the uterus.

Fertilization usually occurs in one of the tubes. The embryo now travels to the uterus, the primary job of which is to sustain development. As it is a muscular organ, it is capable of great stretching. At the distal end of the uterus is the cervix, which attaches to the superior portion of the vagina.

35.6 What is the luteal phase?

The luteal phase starts next with the LH causing the follicle to secrete progesterone instead of estrogen. Progesterone causes the endometrial lining to begin to thicken in preparation for implantation of a fertilized cell. Progesterone inhibits release of FSH and LH. If fertilization does not occur, the corpus luteum, containing the oocyte, dies, which lowers the level of progesterone. Sloughing of the lining begins about the twenty-eighth day of the cycle, resulting in a flow of blood and cellular debris through the vagina.

35.7 What is dysmenorrhea?

Dysmenorrhea is menstrual pain occurring after ovulation for which no cause can be discerned.

35.8 What is an ectopic pregnancy?

An ectopic pregnancy occurs when the fertilized ovum implants in an area other than the uterus.

35.9 What is leiomyomas?

Leiomyomas are smooth muscle tumors of the uterus.

35.10 What is infertility?

Infertility is the inability of a reproductive-age couple to conceive after 12 months of unprotected sexual intercourse.

35.11 What is menopause?

Menopause is defined as 12 months without a menses.

35.12 Why is ovarian cancer a deadly cancer?

Ovarian cancer is the deadliest gynecologic cancer because it is usually advanced before it is detected. There is no proven screening test for ovarian cancer. There are no early signs.

35.13 What is an ovarian cyst?

The most common ovarian cysts are follicular. The egg is enclosed in a follicle as it waits to be expelled monthly from the ovary. When the follicle does not open to allow the egg out or the follicle is not reabsorbed, a benign cyst, a fluid-filled sac, may result.

35.14 What is pelvic inflammatory disease (PID)?

PID is a variety of inflammations and infections of the upper genital tract, which includes the uterus, fallopian tubes, ovaries, and other structures.

35.15 What are common causes of pelvic inflammatory disease PID?

Usual organisms include *Chlamydia trachomatis, Neisseria gonorrhoeae, Escherichia coli,* and *Bacteroides*. Most infections are caused by a mix of bacteria.

35.16 What are trophoblastic neoplasias?

Trophoblastic neoplasias are abnormal cells growing from a shell that forms between the embryo and the endometrium.

35.17 What are the types of trophoblastic disease?

The four disease entities are called hydatidiform mole (partial or complete), invasive mole, choriocarcinoma, and placental site trophoblastic tumor.

35.18 What are choriocarcinomas?

Choriocarcinomas are tumors composed of trophoblasts with bleeding.

35.19 What are placental site trophoblastic tumors?

Placental site trophoblastic tumors are trophoblasts which intrude the myometrium.

35.20 From when is gestational age measured?

Gestational age is measured from the first day of the last menstrual period (LMP).

35.21 What are Braxton-Hicks contractions?

Mild abdominal cramping that is felt from 28 weeks to birth is called Braxton-Hicks contractions.

35.22 What is effacement?

Effacement is the thinning of the cervix.

35.23 What is preeclampsia?

Preeclampsia is a condition that women may get in the latter half of pregnancy. It is pregnancy-induced hypertension.

35.24 What is eclampsia?

Eclampsia are seizures not related to a brain condition.

35.25 How does the second phase of labor end?

The second stage of labor ends with the birth of the baby.

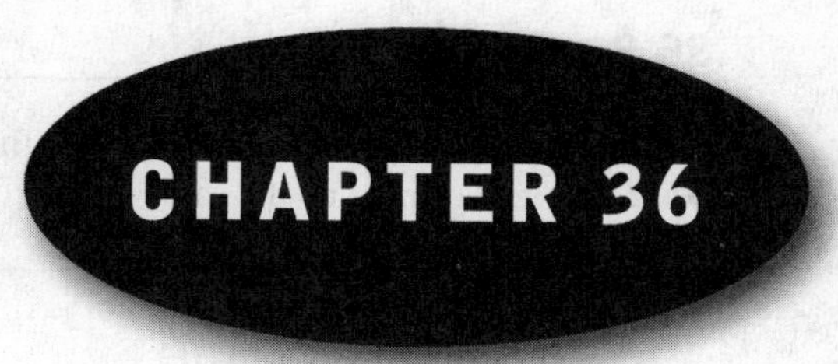

Pain Management

36.1 Definition

Pain is sensed through nerve endings, which are generously spread throughout the internal tissues and the skin. The brain is the only structure without pain receptors. When pain receptors are stimulated, discomfort or pain results, prompting that action be taken to remove the cause of the pain.

The pain impulse travels along sensory fibers of the spinal nerves to the spinal cord and then to the brain, which interprets the degree and source of the pain. The brain can then signal nerve fibers to release chemicals to inhibit pain signals. Some of the chemicals—enkephalins, serotonin, and endorphins—are able to suppress pain signals and provide endogenous pain control.

Visceral pain is pain from an organ secondary to surgery, cramping, ischemia, stretching, or spasms.

Referred pain is the sensation of pain coming from another part of the body than where it actually originates. It is common for heart pain to be felt in the arm. The pain impulses from the heart travel the same circuit as the receptors in the arm, confusing the interpretation in the brain.

Various individuals can experience different levels of pain with the same injury. Researchers have sought to explain this phenomenon. The gate control theory postulates that there is a "gate" in the spine that controls the impulses from the finger on the hot stove to the brain. The brain controls this gate to allow through total or partial signals.

However, the interpretation is based on current emotions, memories, expectations, ideals, and cultural biases. If your mind is busy elsewhere, the pain may be somehow lessened, for example, the Lamaze experience through labor and childbirth. This is one of the more popular pain theories, among others. Emotional pain can produce many symptoms, as varied in their presentation as the etiology of the pain.

Pain scales are useful tools to assess severity of pain and quality of life. They help the patient to accurately assess the pain and the impact it is having. Pain scales often are measured on a Likert scale, from 0 (no pain) to 10 (the worst pain ever).

The Wong pain scale for children uses a happy smiling face to a sad, tearful one. Another useful tool is a pain diary, in which the patient records severity, location, activity at the time, precipitating factors, and what if anything relieved the pain. It is a helpful tool to assess worsening or alleviating pain and reactions to pain medications.

36.2 Acute Pain

Acute pain usually points to an aberration or an illness. It is differentiated from chronic pain by the duration, usually less than 4 to 6 months. Pain nerves are stimulated by pressure, cuts, heat, cold, stabs, surgery, and so on. Other causes include fractures, burns, and bruises.

36.3 Chronic Pain

Chronic pain is lingering pain after identification of etiology of the initial onset. It may be less intense after 4 to 6 months, or may be the same degree of pain.

- Arthritis
- Backaches
- Cancer
- Headaches
- Neurogenic pain
- Psychogenic pain

36.4 Peripheral Neuropathy

This is the degeneration or disease of the peripheral nerves that affect motor and/or sensory nerves. The peripheral nerves include all but the brain and spinal cord. The neuropathies are poorly understood. When peripheral nerves are damaged, the brain becomes confused when processing communication from the damaged nerves.

Pain or numbness may be out of proportion to the damage or may be present where skin and tissue are intact. Peripheral neuropathy may affect motor nerves, sensory nerves, or both. It is often a sequelae (secondary result) of poorly controlled diabetes, autoimmune diseases, hypothyroidism, toxic substances, HIV/AIDS, vitamin deficiencies, alcohol abuse, or some infections.

36.5 Phantom Limb Pain

Pain, mild to severe, felt in the area where an extremity has been amputated, is called phantom limb pain. The nerve endings at the surgical site continue to relay pain signals to the brain. The missing limb could be the result of surgical amputation or trauma.

36.6 Substance Use Disorders

Substance abuse is defined as an irresistable urge for drugs, alcohol, or other substances, including physical, physiologic, and psychological longings, and a need for more and greater dosages to satisfy the cravings.

Abused substances produce euphoria and intoxication, which include changes in mental status, decreased coordination, and slurred speech. Seizures and loss of consciousness are late signs. Usual abused substances include alcohol, club or illegal drugs, and cigarettes. However, food, caffeine, and sex may be included in some definitions.

Research shows a varied set of internal and external circumstances leading to drug abuse. There seems to be a genetic factor involved, as well as environmental and social elements. Individuals may slowly begin a habit for pleasure, depression, hunger issues, weight reduction, societal pressures, or to escape from pressure. Teen use often begins early.

36.7 Drug Addiction

Drug addiction is the chronic overuse and abuse of legal or illegal substances causing interpersonal, social, and family problems. Addiction occurs when the use of the substance causes an abnormal physical or psychological dependence in which sudden discontinuance causes severe trauma. This differs from tolerance, in which the desired effectiveness of the drug diminishes over time.

Larger quantities of the drug must be used to achieve the same effect. Severe addiction is usually characterized by the inability to carry out work requirements, school responsibilities, or family obligations and duties. Some patients who take pain medications other than directed or to achieve a sensation different than pain relief are more at risk for addiction. Addiction is a multifaceted problem caused by peer pressure, genetic factors, social nonconformity, stress, depression, and mental anxiety.

Those who have a family member with an addiction or who have themselves had an addiction in the past are at an increased risk. Societal pressures and environmental pressures can influence the probability of becoming addicted. Research has determined that long-term drug use results in changes in brain function, which increases the compulsion to abuse drugs.

Solved Problems

Pain Management

36.1 What is pain?

Pain is sensed through nerve endings.

36.2 What chemicals can provide endogenous pain control?

Enkephalins, serotonin, and endorphins are able to suppress pain signals.

36.3 What is visceral pain?

Visceral pain is pain from an organ secondary to surgery, cramping, ischemia, stretching, or spasms.

36.4 What is referred pain?

Referred pain is the sensation of pain coming from another part of the body than where it actually originates.

36.5 What is an example of referred pain?

It is common for heart pain to be felt in the arm. The pain impulses from the heart travel the same circuit as the receptors in the arm, confusing the interpretation in the brain.

36.6 What does the gate control theory postulate?

The gate control theory postulates that there is a "gate" in the spine that controls the impulses from the finger on the hot stove to the brain. The brain controls this gate to allow total or partial signals through total or partial signals.

36.7 What is the Lamaze experience?

If your mind is busy elsewhere, the pain may be somehow lessened, for example, the Lamaze experience through labor and childbirth uses relaxation, breathing techniques, and continuous emotional support to direct the mother's mind away from labor.

36.8 What are pain scales?

Pain scales are useful tools to assess severity of pain and quality of life. They will help the patient to accurately assess the pain and the impact it is having. Pain scales often are measured on a Likert scale, from 0 (no pain) to 10 (the worst pain ever).

36.9 What is the Wong pain scale?

The Wong pain scale for children uses a happy smiling face to a sad, tearful one.

36.10 What is a pain diary?

A pain diary is a diary in which the patient records severity, location, activity at the time, precipitating factors, and what, if anything, relieved the pain. It is a helpful tool to assess worsening or alleviating pain and also reactions to pain medications.

36.11 What is acute pain?

Acute pain usually points to an aberration or an illness. It is differentiated from chronic pain by the duration, usually less than 4 to 6 months.

36.12 What are common causes of acute pain?

Pain nerves are stimulated by pressure, cuts, heat, cold, stabs, surgery, and so on. Other causes include fractures, burns, and bruises.

36.13 What is chronic pain?

Chronic pain is lingering pain after identification of etiology of the initial onset. It may be less intense after 4 to 6 months, or may be the same degree of pain.

36.14 What are examples of chronic pain?

Some examples of chronic pain are arthritis, backaches, cancer, headaches, neurogenic pain, and psychogenic pain.

36.15 What is peripheral neuropathy?

This is the degeneration or disease of the peripheral nerves that affect motor and/or sensory nerves. The peripheral nerves include all but the brain and spinal cord. The neuropathies are poorly understood. When peripheral nerves are damaged, the brain becomes confused when processing communication from the damaged nerves.

36.16 What is a result of peripheral neuropathy?

Pain or numbness may be out of proportion to the damage or may be present where skin and tissue are intact.

36.17 What is a cause of peripheral neuropathy?

It is often a sequelae (secondary result) of poorly controlled diabetes, autoimmune diseases, hypothyroidism, toxic substances, HIV/AIDS, vitamin deficiencies, alcohol abuse, or some infections.

36.18 What is phantom limb pain?

Pain, mild to severe, felt in the area where an extremity has been amputated, is called phantom limb pain. The nerve endings at the surgical site continue to relay pain signals to the brain.

36.19 How is phantom limb pain treated?

Health care providers treat phantom limb pain with the same treatment as if the limb was present because the pain is real caused by pain signals from nerve endings at the surgical site.

36.20 What is substance abuse?

Substance abuse is defined as an irresistible urge for drugs, alcohol, or other substances, including physical, physiologic, and psychological longings, and a need for more and greater dosages to satisfy the cravings.

36.21 What results in the use of abused substances?

Abused substances produce euphoria and intoxication, which include changes in mental status, decreased coordination, and slurred speech.

36.22 What is drug addiction?

Drug addiction is the chronic overuse and abuse of legal or illegal substances causing interpersonal, social, and family problems.

36.23 When does addiction to drugs occur?

Addiction occurs when the use of the substance causes an abnormal physical or psychological dependence in which the sudden discontinuance will cause severe trauma.

36.24 How does addiction differ from drug tolerance?

Drug tolerance occurs when the desired effectiveness of the drug diminishes over time.

36.25 What is severe addiction?

Severe addiction is usually characterized by the inability to carry out work requirements, school responsibilities, or family obligations and duties.

INDEX